MW00880563

Holistic Mental Health For The Golden Age

Ulf Haukenes

Copyright © 2018 Ulf Haukenes

All rights reserved.

ISBN: 1542980690
ISBN-13: 978-1542980692

CONTENTS

ACKNOWLEDGMENTS

I WOULD LIKE TO DEDICATE THIS BOOK FIRST AND FOREMOST TO MY AMAZING MOTHER AND BEST FRIEND, SANDRA HAUKENES, FOR NEVER GIVING UP ON ME, WHEN ALL OTHER'S HAD LOST FAITH IN ME, WITHOUT YOU AND YOUR UNWAVERING SUPPORT, THIS BOOK WOULD NOT BE A REALITY AND I WOULD NOT HAVE SURVIVED THE CHALLENGES I WERE GIVEN IN LIFE.

SECOND, I WOULD LIKE TO DEDICATE THIS BOOK TO THE OTHER STRONG WOMEN IN MY LIFE, MY SISTER, EIRIN FOR BEING A STRONG LIGHT OF LOVE AND COMPASSION, IF ONLY MORE WOMEN WERE LIKE HER.

CHAZELLE OWENS, FOR PUSHING ME TO WRITE THIS BOOK.

BRANDY EVES, FOR BEING MY MUSE DURING A DIFFICULT PROCESS AND IGNITING THE FIRE TO FINISH A BOOK THAT HAS BEEN VERY HARD TO WRITE MENTALLY AND EMOTIONALLY AND I COULD NOT HAVE DONE IT WITHOUT YOU,
YOU HAVE BEEN MY ROCK THROUGH THIS PROCESS OF HEALING AND INTEGRATING ALL THESE TIMELINES AND MORE..

THANK YOU ALL   FOR SHARING THIS PASSION FOR OUR INDIVIDUAL AND JOINT PURPOSES IN LIFE TO ASSIST THOSE WHO WALK THIS PATH OF HEALING MIND, BODY AND SOUL, HEYOKA.

I LOVE YOU ALL DEEPLY.

THIRD I WOULD LIKE TO DEDICATE THIS BOOK TO MY
FATHER, FOR BEING THE PERFECT TEACHER FOR ME
TO BECOME WHO I HAVE BECOME AND WHO I AM
BECOMING.
THANK YOU FOR THE ALL THE HEALING WE DID DAD.
WITHOUT ANY OF YOU, I WOULD NOT BE ME AS I AM
TODAY.
THANK YOU, I LOVE YOU.

FOURTH, I WOULD LIKE TO DEDICATE THIS BOOK TO
EVERYONE WHO EVER STRUGGLED WITH MENTAL
HEALTH, PHYSICAL HEALTH AND ALIENATION IN A
VERY ALIEN WORLD, EVERY STRANGER IN A STRANGE
LAND, EVERY OUTCAST OF SOCIETY SEEING
THEMSELVES AS MAD IN PLACE OF THE MAD, MAD
WORLD WE LIVE IN.

YOU ARE NOT MAD, THE WORLD IS MAD.

LAST, BUT NOT LEAST I WOULD LIKE TO THANK MY
MANY AMAZING TEACHERS, GUIDES AND MENTORS IN
LIFE, ARVID M. KARLSEN, JAN DØDERLEIN, OMAR AGIS,
SIGURD EBBESTAD, MARTIN EBBESTAD, MARK
CLOUDFOOT GERSHON, CLAY LOMAKAYU, NIC WHITTY,
MEL BRAND, OWEN FOX, DR. ROBERT MORSE, DR. SEBI
AND DR. ROGER GUNDERSEN,
KRISTIAN THORESEN AND THOMAS SILVER.
THANK YOU ALL FOR YOUR CONTRIBUTION TO MY
LIFE, MY PATH AND PROCESS, YOUR WISDOM LIVE ON
THROUGH ME, AS I PAY IT FORWARD.

HOW TO LOSE YOUR MIND IN A MAD WORLD

I was born into a typical dysfunctional Norwegian middle class family in Norway's oldest city, Tunsberg on a cold Sunday in February. My mother was a "stay at home" mom with 3 jobs on the side, active in sports, great singer and amazing person,
With an ADD diagnose, very energetic, intense and hyperactive as growing up, but when they put her on Ritalin, she changed and became more calm, but with a price. She no longer had the energetic level to keep up with her old self and has ever since been ditsy and misplacing things and many other side effects of use of Ritalin. My father growing up was quite the individual,
He would always sit in his tool shed building things, fixing things and as the computer evolved he would pick apart and put back together every one that came along. Seldom having time for his young family, most of my childhood was spent sitting in stairs waiting for my dad to come to dinner, show up for weekend visits on time or otherwise, wait for him to show up in his own life. He had abandoned his masculine energy, due to his dad disappearing at sea and presumed dead when he was only 9 years old and it made him reject masculine energy, not only within himself, but in his new wife, which held a lot of masculine energy due to her narcissistic mother and father and traumatic events through childhood as a peace maker between two children in grown up suits. If we take one step back in my grandmother's family, We see that she too, was abused and her trauma lead her to be the way she was towards my mother and the same goes on my dad's side, a long line and history of abuse, wounded inner children and narcissism as a result of trauma and abuse. PTSD is something that has also been prevalent in my family, everyone seems to experience traumas early on in life many generations back. My grandfather Werner was a rebel during the second world war and fought for the freedom of our country against the Nazi's, he was also a sailor with many tales of violent episodes at sea and in foreign countries. The man was a respected and loved man of the community, the chief of the power plant and known and loved by all, so they say, but he was also clearly a madman, very fond of drinking a lot when he first drank and a loud and sometimes

even violent man, according to my mother. She had on occasion experienced quite severe and violent episodes within the family dynamic both between her parents and from her father as the mediator and peace maker of her family. One story I remember him telling and I have had told me many times by mom, is a story of my grandpa riding through the desert with a saber cut in his behind, bleeding on a camel until he find a hotel. Whereby entering the hotel and asking for a room is told they have no vacancies in which he replies he will eat all the lightbulbs if he doesn't get a room. This is but a typical example of the madness that lives within my bloodline, my Norse, gipsy, Viking bloodline, so what more to expect?

My grandfather was extremely violent with my mother and my grandmother, something that seems to have created deep seated narcissistic patterns within the family dynamic.
My grandmother abusing her daughters and especially my mom, as she was the black sheep of the family, the narcissistic scapegoat, as the anger, blame and accountability is always transferred and projected, even onto the child rather than be accountable for their own limitations of consciousness.

Something I would come to find during my parent's divorce.
I was already being bullied severely in the streets by peers and older children. Endless number of the kids in the Norwegian suburb projects where war-refugees, immigrants, alcoholics, drug-addicts and other prolific violent minorities were placed,
Had violent and psychopathic tendencies harming animals and the other children for sport. Something I found no interest in growing up, so you would find me in the forest playing or riding my bike and throughout the day, run from these psychopathic bullies and hide or get beat up, so I learned to run and I learned to run fast. My dad was of no use.
He was abandoning his masculine energy after all,
Most of all, he abandoned me and my mom. Daily he abandoned us by isolating himself in his shed, they were always fighting and I guess that was his refuge, I would have needed a refuge myself if I were him, yet he was half to blame for the dysfunctions he was experiencing, something he failed to

realize, since everyone else was always the problem.

My mom has I have come to learn throughout life is no simple woman to live with either. Her anger issues as well as anger transference and projection is quite the mind fuck to try to navigate with a holistic and balanced mind frame even. Lord knows I have tried in my time, but it only ends up in high dysfunctional shouting. Something that was a daily occurrence in our home. If you weren't heard you raised your voice and even revert to toxic name-calling, a program they had both inherited in their childhood as well and would seem to poison our family just as much as the lack of self-love within the family. When I was even younger they were active musicians playing in a blues band, where my mom would get abused in the band by my dad, as she was getting more attention than him and unable to keep the band together, stopped playing and they both slowly lost the song in their hearts.

Mom later tried to sing with another band, but with a demanding job, studies and 2 little children under her arms,

She did not have much time for herself and so her hobbies and self care and love for music slowly faded into the background.

My dad had now gotten a hand out from my grandpa which helped him get a job in an aluminum plant in a nearby city.

So we moved to a suburb projects with heavy energies and a lot of drug and alcohol abuse. I remember one night a big knife went through the wall in my bedroom and there would be a lot of very violent fights right next door. This didn't last long fortunately but the streets were filled with violence and years of severe bullying would send me into my own imagination very often, I even remember astral travelling at night. In the day I would go down to the cliff, with a 300 foot fall and look at the view and imagine flying, at night I would levitate up under the ceiling and run off the cliff and fly out above the city.

In my own little world I created I had a lovely childhood going off into other worlds and in the real world and at home I was having a difficult time with wounded parents not able to make their marriage work and family eventually giving up of helping as my father would find some way of self-sabotaging one way or another. It was an endless of cycle of getting into arguments with the boss, people he worked with and the neighbors and me and my mother always lowering our heads in embarrassment of his very eccentric personality.

I spent most of my early childhood trying to get my father's love, affection and attention somehow, making him drawings and showing him in hopes of approval and praise.

But there never seemed to be enough hours in the day for him to have time for his family, there was always something in need of fixing, repair or otherwise which had to come first, maybe that was the case as we there never seemed to be enough money either, money was always a cause of arguments and the differences in lifestyle often causing violent outbursts where I would sit underneath the stairs and wait for it to cool down. The stairs was a place I would find myself often, often knocking on the wall simply as attempts to communicate normally with my father seemed futile and often ended in knocking and sometimes yelling from a frustrated mother waiting with a warm dinner. I would often console my mother, As I took on an early role of emotional caretaker and confidant, most likely unconsciously from my mother. I would put on shows for my mom to cheer her up, as singing was how we healed in my family, often in the car and I would sing all day in my room. I wanted to be a musician. I remained my mother's emotional little transmuter of energy and helper for years, my dad growing ever more distant day by day, up until the fighting escalated. They entered separation.

During their separation struggles, my sister came into this world and my life got a new bright light little ray of sunshine added to it, I was in love. She was the cutest thing I had ever seen and she quickly became my most favorite thing in the world. She was born purple and had struggled her way into being, a warrior spirit, like her brother. An old soul in a young body. I would take care of her while my mother studied that time and me and my sister bonded deeply during this time, it was a time of more love in my life, yet my father becoming even more distant with me and having a hard time keeping up with care. The fighting would get even worse and my mom eventually threw him out one night.

He immediately got worse, he started drinking and taking pills, threatening to commit suicide and climbing up on the porch yelling and knocking on the doors and windows. Most often not even show up for our weekend-time, when he did, he was either late, drinking and driving or not coming as he was staying with a new girlfriend, which didn't seem to last very long.

I never grew accustom to waiting for my father, I never stopped believing that maybe someday he would change and realize what mattered. But he never did.

My dad had now finally gotten a steady place to live and seeing a therapist seemed to help somewhat, but a weekend we were there he was clearly feeling suicidal again and was sobbing in bed all weekend, I remember taking care of my sister that weekend and watching TV with her, we both even remember the shows we watched that weekend and what I made her.

I was now in the unfortunate place of having to be my parents parent, emotional care-taker, nanny and psychiatrist more often than not. I quickly became more and more depressed, some pictures of that time reveals a boy with a broken will and heart.

And if the problems at home weren't enough my beautiful mom of course soon got a new boyfriend, but this boyfriend had two mentally challenged brothers, in their thirties and late twenties. The two handicapped brothers had a love for cartoons and porn and were fond of cuddling with children, they had a porn stash in a wooden shed by a quarry where one of the brothers would often take me and have sexual conduct with me, without penetration. Often while watching cartoons in the living room and cuddling my belly, his hand would slip down the right side of my waste and stick his fingers under the lining of my pants and he seemed to get excited from teasing me, or the idea of teasing me, but eventually he was. I had not even started ejaculating yet and was already masturbating several times a day, sometimes even hurting my foreskin from masturbating.

I remember it having sometimes even cuts from me violently trying to make sense of my sexual urges and not to say the least my sexual organ and how sexuality fit into life.

By the time I was 11 this all ended, but brother stayed in our lives as my mom's friend and would sometimes babysit my sister, yet I have no memory of him ever harming her.

And she was too young to remember anything she says and I can only hope he never laid a hand on her, as both these brothers are now under a care taking program after many children came forth with allegations and there was a trial. I never stepped forward with my story until later in life, but I had confirmation on the very fogged up memory of the woodened shed, the smelly magazines, the walk to the shed and the many, many, many cartoon cuddles that would be a game of sexual tease where he would cross the boundaries of all acceptable social conduct and fondle with a 9 year old boys sexual organ. Due to the lack of severity in my abuse compared to other children and those I would later come to meet in my self-medication, I would often downplay the abuse and say I was "only" fondled. I didn't remember how he played my mind and made me start abusing myself, but I quickly became a cutter, at 12 I was already an alcoholic. Drinking every weekend with my friends and trying to figure out how to get to first and second base, both my suicidal template and addiction template already set in place as well as a highly distorted sexual template and abuse template. I don't remember the coaxing, however I do remember so much now I am choosing to share my story as I remember it now, in hopes it might help others out there find a path of healing and heart.

This chapter was written in may 2017 and now, September 2018 – This was all I remembered, until recently, but with the help of a very psychic friend and dear brother of mine, Thomas Silver, who tapped into my memories and helped me remember the experiences of severe sexual abuse I had locked away deep within my own psyche. And also stored in both my energy body and physical body as a physical lump in my lymphatic system, which I have since my discovery of it, reduced from the size of a marble to the size of a tiny crystal shard, much like salt or in this case, a sulphur deposit storing trauma layers which can be shown as a brown spot in my eye, also indicating a Sulphur deposit. The rest of my Iris also shows "genetic" weaknesses from the abuse within my DNA, in other words, sexual abuse mutates the DNA, the etheric body, the templates and programs and even the blueprint of the abused, traumatized.

As my mentor Mel Brand says, when a healthy aura is in its optimal state, it is much like a plump grape, but when we experience trauma it becomes shriveled up, much like a raisin.

This in other words explains why PTSD victims and so on have very heightened senses and sensitivity to sensory overload,

Their auras have been weakened, their own personal magnetic field, have been damaged by the abuse or trauma and made the person extremely sensitive to even touch.

Once their etheric body has been stretched and "fluffed up" a little by a good etheric surgeon or energy worker, they will feel sensitive and experience a better way of life, as my direct experience with myself and my clients.

Sexual abuse being one of the hardest traumas to work with as it is in deep layers, it was only until recently after lots of sexual healing with my ex and on my own this past year, I was ready to reveal, the core, have the full wound exposed and then now after 3 decades of having my sexual freedom taken from me, heal it, once and for all.

Thomas, is one of my most amazing soul family "team-members" for this incarnation, he has been with me through some major shifts in vibration, consciousness and been a well of wisdom and compassion during the strangest and most expansive years of my life. He has a way of working, that cannot be denied, as there is just no way he would know how the trees looked, the way it was decorated in the shed, the walk there, his methods of baiting and the way I was dressed.

Thomas asked me, "So, do you have problems receiving oral sex?" And I all of a sudden felt this deep knowing within me,

Tears started flowing, tears of relief, I had been waiting, searching, doing vision quests, harmed myself in my search for my truth, for my memories. As I always remember everything. Always. All the time. Apart from this I have a photographic and extrasensory memory of events and occurrences in my life, something that resulted in a lot of drugs and alcohol in order to cope with my memories, my emotional landscapes and traumas as well as the mad, mad world I found myself in.

But as I am healing I find a lot of clarity and relief in my ability to remember events to such an extent, I can go back and create a lot of healing, by staying with the feelings that come up from the memories, the memories are healed, through various healing techniques and practices that we will look further at later in the book. But I wanted you to know, who I am, my story and what made me into the healer I am today,

It is a story of a very wounded healer, becoming a self-made man and I am not done writing that story yet and what will come from here, might become a book all of its own.

What I want for you is to come with me outside the firmament of the human consciousness bubble and look back at us all.

What I wish for you is to borrow my shamanic view to see illness in a new light, to view your mentally ill close ones in the right light, the light of love, the light of understanding, compassion and most of all, the light of truth. Truth is what we will dive into in this book, my truth, first and foremost, but I think many of you will find your truth and mine to intertwine and unfold like a beautiful divine tapestry of synchronistic delight as you submerge yourself into this book.

It is a book about life, about being human and going mad in a mad, mad world only to realize, you were the only sane one in an ocean of lunatics many times around and especially when around the so called sane ones. So let's take a look at why people sometimes might lose their marbles and the complete and profound joy of finding yourself again, no longer lost at all.

We are born into a mad world. The collective consensus of popular culture is nothing more than a collective psychosis and it is the real dis-ease on this planet. We grow up and into this world highly indoctrinated with a on-taught and bought fascination for celebrities and popular culture figures as if they were gods and non-humans, we feed this collective psychosis through our celebration of these celebrities and the phenomena of mainstream culture through buying music, videos, art and the daily use of mind numbing television, the opiates of the masses. Children growing up knowing every name and title of every useless celebrity and their work and not knowing or even desiring to know themselves. In fact the popular culture and the way in which most of humanity is programmed to demean and hate themselves due to unhealthy body images and expectations programmed into their minds from popular culture. This then turning beautiful children and teenagers into self-loathing, self-destructive easy prey for the many, many industries that feed off of their demise and misfortune. Whether it is the rock and roll artist selling their music with strongly suggestive lyrics of committing suicide or doing drugs, or the artists painting drugscapes or the film director writing drug content promoting material or the famous charismatic actress doing drugs both on screen and off screen, no matter which of these channels of popular culture we are looking at, we can clearly see the individual watching and listening to these same vibrations, becoming indoctrinated and programmed with this very consciousness and mindset, making them easy targets for the more hidden and darker aspects of the popular culture, The drug culture. The drug culture is far more widespread than we would like to believe and it is a cancer on our society and a threat to the evolution of humanity.

And it is a vicious cycle that feeds the oroboruos, biting it's own tail into infinity, as the darker our lives and our planet gets, the more people turn to stimulants and the darker their lives and the planet becomes, increasingly so at an alarming pace.

There has been an expanse of use of stimulants on this planet the past 50 years like never before. And unlike most hippies out there you won't find me promoting the drugs you get on the street any more than you will find me promoting the drugs you get at your local pharmacy. It is all crap to me. One giant toxic pile of crap that only serves to numb the mind and keep the person using it from reaching their full potential. I like to look at it like this, once you are under the consciousness of the stimulant, it is no longer you producing the creative material and so how can you be able to receive the credit of your work, when it is the LSD painting your paintings, or the Cocaine writing your music or the Marijuana producing your poetry or whatever it might be. If you cannot be creative or formidable and excellent without the use of these stimulants or any stimulant then your creativity isn't worth much anyways in my humble opinion. Wanting to use any stimulant, even something as mild as Marijuana (which can be discussed, seeing it's a mild hallucinogen) is actually an escape from the true self and your true vibration and thus it is an attack on the true self, which could be translated to self-hate, lack of love for self or wanting to escape the true state of your being, your natural vibration and frequency. Any over use of toxins is not something a spiritually mature individual would do, as spiritual maturity is being accountable as a custodian of creation, meaning your mind, body and spirit and your surroundings. Use of strong stimulants that alter your vibration, even caffeine as it is highly toxic to the endocrine system, sends signals to the cells in your body that you are not good enough and not worthy of your own as well as other's love. Abuse is abuse, as simple as that. If you cannot go even a day, a week or a month without any person, place or thing, then you are most likely addicted and suffer dependency and you need help to heal your inner child and come into balance from within.

As long as we keep seeking external gratifications and rewards and using unhealthy coping mechanisms to deal with ourselves, others and life in general we will keep adding layers and layers of trauma upon trauma to our healing process and most do this throughout a whole lifetime not knowing how they sabotage their own life and make their lives living hell in the process of coping with the hell they are experiencing from within and creating more of in their external experience of life.

If we can heal our internal experience of life, our thought processes and our emotional landscapes, we come to find spiritual maturity as a result of this healing. We grow up mentally and can control our minds, much more easily and we can surf the waves of our emotions a lot better and deal with life in a whole new way, far away from the toxic coping mechanisms we have been programmed with from parents, peers and popular culture.

The healing of the inner child is fundamental to this process of spiritual maturity and without healing the inner child, we never really grow up, no matter how old our body may seem, we are still a child and very much immature when faced with challenges or having expectations unmet, we resort to temper tantrums or even violence as means of expressing our dismay or having our way in an attempt to getting our needs met etc.

I am not against either use of drugs, emotional and spiritual immaturity.
I am not in opposition of any consciousness or mindset, however I am pro-active in the expanse of awareness and shedding awareness on consciousness in the way it is lacking in my honest opinion.
I see so many promote stimulants and it's use and the likes of psychedelic advocates such as Joe Rogan, who in my eyes look like nothing more than a teenager who just took LSD and think they have it all figured out.

Same goes for many musicians coming out of popular culture, very unhealthy programs and patterns being displayed in most lyrics and expressions of art. These are very spiritually immature individuals in the high seat of popular culture indoctrinating our youth with a very unhealthy mindset. These keys are nothing more than keys and not a lifestyle choice and they should be revered and respected as such. And they are equally toxic as the toxic society we find ourselves living in. And clearly not the solution to the future of mankind. The lack of respect people have for their own minds as well as these substances is very disconcerting and alarming to someone who has lost their minds at one point in life due to lack of respect for both. It is an easy way to insanity in an already insane society, based in deeply psychotic delusions that are under consensus accepted as reality that shapes and forms every mind of every child from the day the start learning their first words. Everything is a program on this planet, the thing is, what do you choose to program yourself with. The vibration a word holds here on planet earth due to your definition of the word, the definition you most likely have been programmed to define it with, would not hold the same vibration of this planet, it's very meaning would be something different on another planet. This is how easily we are programmed on this planet, with definitions and imagery associated with words and phrases I could do something as simple as say the word "Camel" and you see a camel in your mind's eye, this is how simple it is to program an individual on this planet especially with set definitions to words and phrases. Someone who has not been programmed with earth definitions would not see a camel in their mind's eye, but something entirely different or maybe nothing at all.

Then to take this a step further, now look to the vibrations, consciousness and energy of whatever it is you part-take in, be it your friends, the books you read, the music you listen to, the movies you watch, the art you love or whatever medium it is that you part-take in leaves an imprint of its consciousness in yours and you are more and more a product of your environment and less and less the true you, the pure consciousness you were when you were born into this mad, mad world. This is how simply we are indoctrinated, programmed and patterned from child birth and throughout our lives. Every little incision making us less and less who we truly are and more and more a product of the society we inhabit and make ourselves prone to programming from. It is no wonder so many are losing their minds in this world these days, they grow up in a semi psychotic household with a full blown psychotic culture filled to the rim with toxicity and mental illness masked in popular culture and the mainstream consensus of what is our reality. I remember fairly early on, thinking to myself how everything was wrong down here, even the way my parents loved each other and the way my friends acted and "loved" me. It was all very lacking and toxic, few had the heart I had, few shared willingly, few gave without needing anything in return. By the time I was 9 I had shut down my heart a lot in order to belong with the crowd, by the age of 9, I had given up, I have found pictures of myself from that time in my life and I look like caged, tormented and beaten down animal robbed of all will to live and love. I had finally been crushed by the weight of the world and how it all works down here. My parent's divorce was a tiny bump in the road, compared to my grandfather's death and the sexual abuse I was now experiencing. Overstepping my boundaries and tainting my ability to receive pleasure. Soon most of my power of love would be turned into fear and hate. I quickly became a suicidal young man, having seen my father in a suicidal state after my parent's divorce also programmed me with a very deep victim mentality, if things became hard, I could always kill myself.

Even though I knew very well, that my parents were not grown up's at all,

How could they be so immature and fight and whine and moan like little babies? How could they not handle life? They were clearly not wiser than I, they clearly did not have it together or understand more than I did.

Something was wrong on this planet and I swore to figure it out.

Deep contemplation and meditation is something I always was prone to,

Drifting away into the deep questions of the cosmos and mankind were daily activities for me at a very young age. I loved reading history books, old mythologies and war history at 3-4 years old I can remember the smell of them at my grandparent's house still. Eventually they were all given to me. I went on to get a typewriter from my grandpa and an old English dictionary as I wanted to write English lyrics and essays at 5-6. My dictionary and notebook were steady companions. I was determined to write rock music and in American English of course. Norwegian sounded weird to me, it always did. A hard language to sing in, even for a Norwegian, hard to make it sound lovely as the old-germanian languages do not flow as easily as the English language does. Music would be the way I was to be programmed the most. I wanted to be a rock star, I wanted the hot women and the feeling of being on stage, conducting all those energies and being at the center of attention, where bands like W.A.S.P., KISS and the likes were my main-programmers, womanizing and sexual programming being at the heart of this music, I can say I was programmed with sexual distortion fairly early on, at 4 years old I was already certain what I wanted to be in life and it was not a fireman, it was a rock star.

Our children are indoctrinated and programmed in this way

daily from TV, media, Music and Mainstream Popular Culture. And through this programming they will lose their true self and become products of society.

Infected with the worst disease known to man, the collective consensus known as culture, the cancer of the heart and mind of every man, woman and child of this planet. The real reason your sons and daughters hate themselves and want to die. The real reason they are unhappy and wanting to do drugs, they are programmed to do so, they are programmed to want to do that which is illegal as just one more step to rob them off their spirit and ultimately also their freedom. The very machinery that is programming them is the very machinery that benefits from their demise, the Hollywood machinery, the music industry, Television. Making our children want to become movie stars, rappers, gangsters, drug lords, porn stars, strippers, rock stars and other toxic and delusional programs they are programmed with through the media machinery. Then of course we have the other equally toxic programming from channels such as Disney and the romantic love template industry, promoting prince charming, white picket fences, 2 and a half children, 2 cars, a cabin, a boat and expensive vacations to far away tropical regions to modulate the perfect family. With no less toxic outcomes than the drugged up variety we took a look at earlier. Only this time, the drugs do not come from your streets, but from your friendly neighborhood drug dealer, the allopathic doctor, peddling you drugs for every malnutrition that over time has become an imbalance in your mind, body and spirit. A pill for every condition, yet no cure for anything but curiosity. Your curiosity will be cured with mind numbing chemicals to make sure you don't ask any questions that might set your mind free. A depression becomes suicidal tendencies from the side effects of your depression pills. You are now worse off than you initially were and can be given more "medication" to make sure you become a perfect swing door patient in need of their services. How many pills in total is prescribed for your specific household?

In my time it was about a bag. A bag of pills for a few months. With 5 pills for 5 various conditions and then 3 pills for the side effects of these 5 other pills. I knew something was up, something did not feel right. I had all these pills and medications and I was still not getting any better, only getting worse and worse by the day. So I decided to come off the pills, I stopped taking them all, something I do not recommend professionally, talk to your doctor about weening yourself off slowly from these strong "medications", as quitting cold turkey may give powerful side effects and be counterproductive to your healing process or in worst case scenario, kill you, as that is how strong they are and how much they disrupt natural hormone levels and chemistry in the body.

A regular anti-depressant has side effects such as suicidal tendencies, so please be careful both with usage and coming of these chemical cocktails prescribed from your doctors.

To truly come back to true health and wellbeing, a holistic approach will be necessary, as with allopathic healing with medication you first have to heal from your ailment and then you will have to heal from the use of medication. If you use a holistic approach to healing you won't have to heal from the side effects of said medication. Changing our lifestyle is a must on the path to healing if we are to live a consciously happy and thriving life.

There are no short cuts to complete and lasting health. For me the journey back to health took me almost a decade from the moment I decided to come off the medication to the radiant health I have today from the inside out. My organs, hormones and over all wellbeing took many turns and sometimes I took 3 steps back before taking 2 steps forward again, only to find myself having to start all over again from scratch as it wasn't always easy eating healthy when I had few people around me eating healthy as well.

Food addiction and bad habits alongside expensive organic foods and cheap processed foods everywhere are two of our greatest adversaries to true health and wellbeing. There isn't much else to do, than to actually invest long term in healthy living or we pay the price through illness and falling back into disease and suffering. So the extra money we spend on healthy eating, herbal supplementation truly pays off in the long run, something I and most of my health conscious friends who have healed severe illness are a living embodiment and example of today. Even when it comes to food we live in an insane world, truly. Food-like products are masked as food for children filled to the rim with chemicals from processes that eliminates all nutrition from the "foods" we are exposed to from birth.

Minerals and Vitamins are long gone by the time it hits the shelves in our stores in order to preserve shelf life for as long as possible.

People are more addicted to flavors and textures than they are wanting actual nutrient rich foods that charge their cells and feeds their light and body. Food is supposed to carry frequency and energy, in other words, it needs to contain light in order to actually spark your cells alive like the ignition in the engine of your car, your food is meant to ignite and spark life into your cells and make you come alive. If your food is dead, overly processed and lacking in nutrients, it is not food, but empty fillers like most of the programs in your T.V. (Tell-Lie-Vision), mindless crap to keep you contained within entertainment. You enter containment. Take for example the music on today's CD's, you have 2 hit songs and the rest bland, tasteless crap to fill a need for the consumers and we all buy it and it is the same with our food, you have flavor and toxic addictive additives masking the lack of nutrients. It is nutrients your body craves once you become healthy, not flavor, a need for artificial flavor is actually a result of our food-addiction and the many "spices" and additives put in our food-like "food".

There is very little substance to actually feed your mind, body and spirit in any mainstream consumption, whether it be food, clothing, entertainment or otherwise, we see very little quality over quantity and mass production made for mass consumption, but putting cheaply made food into your precious body is the same as telling your body you do not appreciate it and thus do not love it. Self-love is eating right. Self-love is maintaining your vibrant life-force aiming for longevity and a good and healthy life.

Once more we return to spiritual accountability, spiritual accountability means loving your mind, body and spirit enough to want them in their true state, in their original vibration, unaltered by toxic stimulation from bad eating, drugs and other easy ways out from coping with existence in a healthy manner.

You see in our search for spiritual sovereignty, we will at some point come to the realization that anything that does not serve us, will have to be removed for the purpose of full mastery of our existence.

Full spiritual sovereignty means not going to the doctor handing over accountability for your own health to a complete stranger, but being 100% accountable for your own wellbeing at all times. This means you will have to learn how to communicate with your body, learn how to read your own body's language. Learn how to control your mind, feelings and energy.

This means you will eventually have to stop altering your mind and natural vibration daily with substances, be it something as "mild" as marijuana or coffee or sugar or even chemical laced processed foods for comfort. I am of course not talking about medicinal use or occasional recreational use, but too much of even a good thing, becomes a bad thing when we look at it holistically and with a close look at the endocrine system which struggles to produce enough dopamine f.ex with excessive cannabis use. Now I love this plant and recommend it's use for healing and treating a variety of imbalances, but I also have great respect for this medicine as it has been my most trusted plant ally as well as my very harsh mistress, as the spirit of cannabis is a jealous female as my Toltec mentor Mark Cloudfoot Gershon says, which I do agree on. She has claimed a lot of time, space, money and even relationships in her time and learning how to balance my use of this plant ally has been detrimental to all my creative and professional endavours.

Even too much cannabis will deplete our system of nutrients, hormones and put us out of balance, a diagnosis known as "Cannabinoid hyperemesis syndrome", is a condition that can occur with copious cannabis use and is characterized by recurrent nausea, vomiting, and crampy abdominal pain.

Having trouble eating without the use of cannabis in the morning can be a sign of this condition and I would strongly suggest lowering your dosages and use.

I believe we can learn to master our relationship to any substance once we learn to master our relationship to ourselves and the universe and develop a pro-noia where you believe the universe is working in your favor. To then view the plants that show up for you as also messengers of the cosmos and what your body needs as well, is a very hermetic and herbalist way of viewing plant medicine and medicine in general, but is the way all our native people and ancestors have communicated with nature and the flora and fauna for millennia.

We have always had this relationship to the cosmos and nature and there is a revival of all our ancient cultures currently on a global scale and it is putting us back into integral symbiotic relation with mother earth. To learn how to see what shows up for you frequently can mean a world of difference as nature heals us a lot faster than these synthetic medicines from the pharmacopeia of modern society.

Be aware of when you use something or even someone as a crutch/coping mechanism and tool and when it is becoming detrimental to your health and well being to change your habits. Going to the doctor and getting a prescription won't change the fact of the matter that you need to change your lifestyle, you will only prolong your own time in healing.

Anything can become a drug or an escape from our true vibration and food is certainly no different than stimulants. Be it people, places, events or things being used as a means to escape one's own true self and true state of being and vibration. Anything can become an escape from self. Many use music, TV and even internet as a means to escape their true state of being, their own thoughts is the enemy, their own feelings is the enemy and they use external stimulation as the remedy. People are like drugs to them, clingy and co-dependent. TV and music are like drugs to them, they cannot go without stimulation of image and sound or they are forced to look at themselves, forces to sit with their own thoughts and feelings. These people are at war with their natural state, they are running from their true self, programmed to deceive themselves, programmed to hate themselves,

Unable to be in themselves, they seek any means necessary to escape learning about themselves, chances are if they stopped for only a little while enough to actually feel and listen, they would come to find how truly beautiful they are and stop running from themselves and end the escape from self and come into full spiritual sovereignty. In fact, there is no other way into full spiritual maturity, than through the silence of mind. There is no short cut to ascension of mind, body and spirit. There is no transmutation and complete alchemy without going through the inner.

If we continue to escape going within, we will never find our treasure, our inner riches and sanctuary, where there always will be peace to be found.

No matter the circumstance, as only state of being matters once we have found our inner peace, it is brought with us everywhere.

I invite you now before we end the first chapter to take 30 minutes to an hour, to sit in silence with your mind, body and spirit.

Place your left hand on your heart center,
Place your right hand on your solar plexus (the belly button)

Take 3 deep breaths.
In through the nose.
All the way down into your abdomen.
Slowly out the mouth.
Like you are blowing out a candle.
This is called a Prana Breath.
This is your access to universal life force.
It is free. And it is deeply healing.
This technique was shown to me by my higher self in my "psychosis" or kundalini syndrome.
And it is a way to align the heart center and the emotional center for the purpose of emotional healing.

Use this technique whenever you feel the need to align yourself and come back to center and your own peace. It is my gift to you, the reader as a thank you for having chosen to read my book, whether you have purchased my book or borrowed it from a friend or loved one.

You have chosen the road to healing and for that I commend you and give you my deepest blessings. Close your eyes for a moment and tap into the gratitude I have for you for choosing to heal yourself and thus heal the world.

And thank you for deciding to read my thoughts on what causes mental illness in this world in my humble opinion from what has been my experience throughout life, both from observation and personal experience.

THEY ARE COMING TO TAKE ME AWAY HI-HI

We live in a world where murder and violence on Tell-Lie-Vision is more socially acceptable than two people making love and showing each other how much they love, adore and appreciate one another. This is how sick society actually has become. Ethics and norms are in desperate need of revision and upgrade in this psychotic rape culture we live in.

We rape the planet we live on from all natural resources and we rape our mother's, sisters, daughters, brothers and sons. Sexual abuse is so wide-spread on this planet out of the 10 women I have been in a relationship with, only 1 was not sexually abused or molested in some way, shape or form. We are prone to violation and violence on a daily basis, from media, from entertainment and art, we are constantly being desensitized from any and all directions within our confounds of society to not be outraged by the violence we are subjected to on a daily basis. Why you may ask?

Because the war machine is another machinery that greatly benefits from our desensitization and it is a trillion dollar industry that also in the end supports the drug industry on both sides legal and illegal, it supports the other trillion dollar industries such as Gold, Oil and Diamonds. (G.O.D.)

It is this God it seems the many nations leadership truly believes in and the money they make are smeared in the blood of our young and innocent, long before they ever even find their way into the military. Money and resources are deeply imbalanced on this planet. We have more than enough to go around for everyone, yet the rich get richer and the poor get poorer by the second. We are living in a time of over-population, that is true, there is no way the planet will be able to sustain the increase of population the way it is expanding beyond sustainability. And the only way we could turn this around, is if resources were better shared amongst us all.

I awoke to these truths and many others in 1997 at the age of 18 and it crushed my spirit. I realized we, humanity were sawing off the branch we are sitting on and pouring toxins down the well we drink from.

I quickly became extremely depressed as my sensitive nature had a very hard time living with this fact and realized I had awoken to a world of sleepers. And at the time there was no online community as the many have today, there were few to talk about these things with or even come together with to find solutions to issues I saw needed addressed.

I was alone, I felt abandoned and left behind by my creator, how in the world could I be so alone in seeing these things which were so apparent to my ancient eyes. I was devastated, I tried reaching out through my art, my music in hopes to reach like-minded or to have my message reach out to the masses in hopes to awaken them to the truths I saw.

But I had become lost myself, lost in drug abuse as a means to cope with the atrocities I witnessed all around me. I quickly fell back asleep.

Searching still for higher levels of consciousness, but not in the right manner, I was still not fully opened in my heart, I was way too angry with humanity for their violence towards our mother earth, I hated them so deeply I would have easily blown up society had I had access to such devices. They were pests and a virus in my eyes and they needed to be washed away so mother earth could become a jewel once more as she was meant to be. She is holy and sacred and the way they treated her was in no way sacred, nor holy, it was rape and violation, much like everything else on this planet conducted by humankind.

I quickly started losing my mind to the anger, to the outrage and little by little I became an antisocial pessimist bordering towards sociopathic tendencies, much like most of my peers and those who see the truths too early without the heart to back it up.

A third eye awakening without the spiritual maturity and heart center to back it up, will raise a fury in most men only the legions of war can match.

To no surprise I was soon to be going in and out of emergency rooms, mental facilities and nights spent in jail.

I was now become a public enemy, daily harassed by police and authority due to my anti-social ways and regularly visited the institutions linked to these organizations in attempts to subdue my violent nature to little or no avail as the more they harassed me and the more I was tormented the more like an animal I became, something we see mirrored on a grand scale within our society. The war on drugs and the war on alternative thinking and alternative living breeds a great contempt and dismay amongst the young ones making them soldiers in a war for consciousness that takes lives daily, whether we like to admit it or not. Our children are cannon fodder for a war on consciousness and it is our responsibility as elders , parents and conscious beings to inform and educate them to work for a more sustainable way of living, loving and thriving on planet earth, which is my incentive for writing this book, as much as it is assisting in the healing of mental illness on a collective scale, it is also a call to change of the collective psychosis and how to heal and teach our younger generations for a more sustainable future. We can all play our part, by being the right person, saying the right thing at the right time to the right people in dire need of a wholesome mind and sounding board so we can all see a better future for our planet.

We are all in this together after all and I for one, would love to see change on this planet before I leave it in a better condition than when I came here.

There is no escaping the fact that our children are in need of better leaders, whether they are politicians, musicians or other leaders, we do not need better followers, we need better guides, sounder leaders, then we will see better followers as well, but someone has to take the first step.

Will   you   be   one   of   the   first?

I sure hope so, I hope this book will be enough for you reading my words to realize the power you hold, to be just what this planet needs, in every moment of your day you can do the right thing, say the right thing and be the right person, or not...It is all up to you. Only you can change you and your own surroundings and your experience of life starts with you.

Healing the world starts at home, it starts with us, the individual, not the masses, the masses will heal as a result of each person, each home healing.

And so this book is a call to all parents, it is a call to all teachers, all brothers and sisters to be the role model the younger ones need.

The elders of this planet also will learn from your ways and your being if you embody the change you wish to see yourself.

Do you wish to see change? That is the question and the answer is quite simple, you have to be that which you seek, we do not change the world by telling others how to live or how to be, we change it by being the change we wish to see, we change it by changing ourselves. This is true spiritual accountability.

I was once a rebel, locked up in a mental ward with multiple diagnosis, severely ill in mind, body and spirit, but I chose to change, I chose a better life for myself and my loved ones and by choice I made it so.

And you can too, the power to change is all within your hands, within your grasp, but you must reach for it, you must make the choice and it is a daily one. I do not believe that we are addicts forever like A.A or N.A. speaks of, I believe we have the power to heal from our addictions and become sovereign, I believe we have the power to heal from our madness, from our diseases, from our feelings of lack and powerlessness and become sovereign in our state of being, by finding and loving our own, true state of being. Unaltered, without stimulation, without instant gratification.

I know one thing for certain and that is if I with my diagnose of Schizoid personality disorder, hearing other people's thoughts, "hearing" their intentions and intent and hearing voices telling me to kill myself, if I can heal, with all these deep torments and more, then you can too and I will tell you all the secrets to my own healing and process in this book and give you all the tools you need to create a daily healing agenda to get back the control of your own mind, body and spirit, completely holistic and 100% natural. But first I will tell my story, my journey into mental illness and the various treatments and medications I was given and the effects it all had on me and how I discovered ways to cope with the feeling of constant fight or flight energy surging through my mind, body and spirit 24/7 and the guidance I got from my higher self and guides along the way to make it easier for me to stay within the private hell I had created for myself with the help of a mad society, a broken health system and the fact that I was always falling between two chairs. Never being sober enough to receive help and never being mentally stable enough to find peace to not seek stimulants in order to calm me down find healing and solace for my wounds or even find balance enough to have a good and decent life. Always having this voice in the back of my head, telling me I was not good enough, I was not what society wanted and I was not man enough according to the toxic macho ideal we see being programmed into the hearts and minds of young men in our society today. It just never felt right, hardening up never felt natural to me, not expressing my emotions and showing my true feelings was just not an option for me, so I was thought of as imbalanced, deemed weak by a sick and toxic society, not realizing that it was them there was something wrong with and not my precious soft and sweet self. I grew anxious very early, I was an alpha male, but I was not prone to the competitive nature of my peers, I saw them as brute and ignorant, which they by all means were, yet they most likely were suffering as much as I , if not more from being hardened up, unable to communicate their emotional landscapes with such clarity and lucidity as I were. Yet I was the one made to feel different and strange and it made me feel crazy, this growing feeling of being different, weird, "something wrong with", in need of fixing made me look within myself in search for what could be done to mend me. It was like a slow landslide daily pushing me closer and closer to the edge of sanity, until I eventually snapped and my imbalances got the best of me. I was to experience many years of run-ins with the law and mental health care, therapy, counseling, medication and a depressed young man in his early 20's was put on anti-depressants and sedatives to fight a growing feeling of alienation and being deeply misunderstood and judged for my thinking, my feelings and my personality. Personality disorder they diagnosed me eventually, chronic suicidal was another and "addict" when in all actuality I was a young man with deep wounds of abandonment, severe bullying and soul torment from seeing things from a higher perspective than most of my fellow men. Occasionally I would find music and art that expressed the ways I thought and on a much rare occasion a person to talk to that felt the same way and saw things as dark as I did. I lost sight of the light in this world, unable to see the good for all the bad and dark ways of society and mankind. It overtook me, put me in a deep rooted anger, hate and my suicidal feelings grew stronger and stronger both from the malnutrition and drug abuse I was trapped in, but also the medication from the doctor making it even worse and my brain and body eventually so chemically imbalanced from all the ongoing and increasing factors in my life.

I was on the highway to hell, with nothing stopping me as I had not a care in the world. I had a hard time caring for anyone as I was unable to relate to anyone, even my family and friends. They did not understand me and the only one that did understand me, was one of my friends parents, who was a psychiatric nurse with addiction problems and an immense love for literature, music and art. We quickly became friends and he was my life-line into reality for many years as I grew more and more unstable from my substance abuse and medication alongside a sever lack of understanding and utilization of nutrition. All I cared about was my escape from my emotional and mental state, all I wanted was to slip into a psychedelic coma or a momentary pill induced coma topped with cannabis.

Cannabis was my daily drug, it was my mistress, my one true love, but she is a jealous mistress and will not let anyone or anything else take the place of being number one in your life once she has taken a hold of you. She, Mary Jane, comes first, before family, before friends and yes, even your own health and well-being, your ambitions quickly fading into the smoke and mirrors of the foggy haze she creates.

She demanded all my money, all my time and all my love, having relationships became increasingly hard over the years and I was as good as married to this substance and she would not let me go, she made me even more depressed, more paranoid, more suicidal as she alienated me further and further into isolation and I let her, she was my one true friend, the one that was always there. She would listen, when nobody else cared, she would give me peace, calm me down when nothing else would. Eventually I became resistant and needed more and more and eventually she was like decaf, hardly working and I needed more pills and harder substances to find my piece of mind. In the end the cocktails were so extensive they would have put down a horse they told me, which was not far from the truth.

The dosages were eventually suicidal and would put me in too many near death experiences to count, resuscitated and brought to the E.R. endlessly and many times it was deliberate and anger my first reaction upon waking back up to life. Life was my curse, I tried so many ways to die and some might say it was cries for help, but after a while it is no longer a cry for help but shouting for death, screaming inside for relief and in the end you only hate that which keeps you alive or brings you back to life.

I lost friend after friend in the process, either to suicide, overdose or from overstepping their boundaries and disrespecting them, but mostly from my endless inner and outer dialogues of the darkness I perceived in this world or the pain I experienced in between manic humor and laughter and melancholic musical expressions I kind of forced them to listen to as they were my only sounding board. Some of which was great work, most of which were trashy, druggy productions on bad equipment. But in the end I probably had 20 out of 200 productions that were good, but messed up every chance to produce with a good producer due to my drug habit and eventually my hard drive collapsed and 7 years of music was lost. I lost faith, I stopped producing electronic music and went back to slamming on my guitar alone, jamming by myself and channeling music onto a cassette recorder. But the passion for writing music quickly faded again into the drug abuse and depression and the longing to play with a band, lead me to desert my arts. I no longer drew, painted, wrote or played, I only wanted to watch mindless movies and eat junk food and pop my prescription pills. Sugar had now become a new addiction, due to it's effect alongside the valiums and my teeth and weight was to suffer immensely.

Nutrition was still something I did not care much about,

I only wanted flavor and I still did not care if I lived or died and my diet mirrored this sentiment. I was on a fast track to a breakdown, both mentally, emotionally and now also physically declining. I had gone from weighing 99 pounds at my lowest with anorexic and bulimic tendencies to 300 pounds with emotional eating, but gained 60 pounds within 3 months from mostly the pills alone and once I had gained that much weight I no longer cared about my appearance and even less about my well-being than ever. My time mostly spent watching neutral and feel good movies and trying to find music that did not trigger my addiction and make me want to do drugs again as well as learning how to find peace with my new existence.

Sugar quickly became a new crutch and addiction and I started smoking more cigarettes than I had been before. New addictions are often found and utilized when we give up old ones and old patterns are often continued with new forms of expression and addiction. Needless to say the sugar addiction started wreaking havoc on my energy, my hormone levels and kept making me increasingly sick. This was most likely the time I started creating candida within my body as I had not had much in-take of sugar or any food for that matter for a really long time, up until this point drugs and chemicals were my main consumption with occasional good nutrition every 3-4 days when I arrived back home at my mother's house in a futile attempt to gather strength and come down from the chemical cocktails I took part in at the house parties and the EDM scene. I had been severely under nourished for years and was now very malnourished lacking fundamental nutrients over time, which in my eyes is a breeding ground for a spiritual awakening gone wrong. I am certain without a tiny percentage of doubt that if I had been taking better care of myself, my kundalini awakenings later on would have not resulted in kundalini crisis and kundalini syndrome, or psychosis if you will and put me through such hard-ship. Everyone will at some point have a spiritual awakening on this planet at this time as the energies are pushing us through spiritual evolution, so whether you have had a kundalini awakening or not, realizing these facts may come to serve you either now or at a later point in your soul's evolution. I will come back to this later in the book.

HEAVILY MEDICATED AND HEAVILY MEDITATED

What I fear most when it comes to western medicine is their complete lack of education when it comes to nutrition and their complete lack of concern for the side effects the medication has on their patients. They are paid by the various corporations that produce the so called medicine and so their trust and integrity and not to mention morals is highly questionable.

There is little to no concern and from my perspective a great deal unconsciousness from the medical community when it comes to how they perceive toxic synthetic "medicine" as something that will heal the ailments the patients are suffering from. And with a rising number of forceful medicating through mental health wards and psychiatric evaluations in the many institutions, there is little many of us could say when being placed lawful force on our choice of healing and many if not most of us being mere guinea pigs for controversial and experimental drugs. With many of us ending up with severe side effects and in some cases death.

They are playing Russian roulette with the lives of young people in order to make money from a trillion dollar industry that is heavily marketed and pushed down your throat by force if you so should happen to be unfortunate enough to struggle with mental health issues. This is a raising concern and my personal experience and incentive for writing this book, I was on the receiving end of this treatment and I was lucky enough to find my way out of this political, medicinal and societal maze construct known as western medicine. Yes, I do believe in rare cases surgery is needed and medication needed with great scrutiny upon having tried all other possibilities, but I believe we tend to listen far too easy and put far too much trust and faith in someone else to know what your body is telling you.

This is why I am hoping to raise awareness and offer accountability of your own mind, body and spirit back to you, through my understanding, experience and wisdom gained through blood, sweat and tears over two very long decades. It sure did not come easy, so my hope is that as many as possible will buy my book and if you happen to read this book and have gotten it for free and it is serving you, may you please consider donating a even a little amount to support me in this work so I can keep writing helpful material to those who are struggling with what most likely both you are or have been struggling with and when you have read this book yourself, share it with someone else, so that they too may be set free from the confounds of western medicine and the tyranny of health care.

Eventually I got to a point where I was so mentally unstable, they locked me up in a mental ward for 3 months and this would be the tipping point of both my reason from unreasonable treatment as well as synchronistic events unfolding further to awaken me to the truths of the universe. In 2007 I was sentenced to 3 months in prison due to my struggles with my instability and I was too mentally ill to serve my time, yet too drugged up for treatment, but somehow was lucky enough to find a double diagnose mental facility that would treat both my mental illness as well as my addiction. I went through substantial cognitive therapy and it would prove to be very helpful, however the medication I was given would prior and during would prove to be very damaging. Side effects that would give me restless legs syndrome, increase my weight and lose my hair (alopecia universalis) and make me very tired. However there were some amazing therapists there that would help me lead me back to myself through meditation and a common interest in spirituality and shamanism. And others that were very active and would lead me back to hormonal health through exercise and give me healthy habits that I would take with me in the coming years. Lifting weights now made me confident and more fearless and I was growing large in every way, not just in terms of fat, but muscle mass and in spirit. Exercise and eating better would prove to be fundamental keys to thriving more both mentally and emotionally and also now physically more than I ever had in my entire life. The only thing was these medications they kept giving me, they were stunting my growth and expansion and they were changing them out, testing one after the other in hopes to find something that would work for my diagnosis they said, but they all came with side effects that would prove to be worse than my actual condition. I came home from the minimal security mental facility and within a few month's time had my kundalini awakening that summer in the month of may. The synchronicities had grown and become too much to deal with and would make me feel chased, under surveillance by all of creation and on the radio songs would play that seemed to taunt me and the TV play shows that would seem to taunt me, the synchronicities were tormenting me and making my mental state worse and worse. It kept increasing to such a point my body was so full of fight and flight energy and I went into full blown psychosis, or what I later came to understand, kundalini crisis with kundalini syndrome. I ended up having 5 very rough days and nights where I eventually ended up spending 48 hours trying to kill myself, with cutting my wrists up and emptying my body of blood into a bucket after having tried to drown myself in the lake frantically and beating myself unconscious with an iron rod from my weight lifting equipment I had gotten to get in shape after my stay in the ward. I ended up in the ER that morning after, almost drained of blood and beaten to pulp by own hand, I was desperate to escape life and this energy I was feeling. With the incompetent alternative health practitioner as well as the incompetent western doctors I ended up so imbalanced the only solution to my troubles was death, no shamanic understanding was present in or around me and so I was lead to believe I was going mad from the people around me as well as so called professionals. Needless to say, the power of suggestion was so strong I eventually believed them and went full blown crazy. Losing all trust in myself and my inner voice, which actually was guiding me to ground my energy out on the lawn and to keep my energy light and the colors around me bright, preferably light or white. But the voices of those around me and the doctors were louder and had me believe I was going mad. Now I later have come to realize this is nothing more than a spiritual awakening that many if not most on the planet will go through at some point in more or lesser degrees and I am pioneering in this sense and am lucky to be alive here today to assist and tell you my story,

31

so that you or someone you love, might not have to experience what I did. After my suicide attempt I realized I was not allowed to leave the planet, not by my own hand, I felt cursed, cursed to live in a private hell. A very lonely isolated existence drenched in symptoms of kundalini syndrome, which the medical community labeled schizo-type personality disorder, agoraphobia and a deep depression, whereby my dog, my family and the sanctuary I had created for myself were my only remedies and it kept me alive having this space by myself. Being placed in disability and receiving money while in therapy exposing myself to the various things I feared slowly and surely in my own time would also prove to be very beneficial.

I was extremely lucky to be living in a socialist country where I could reap the benefits of the social structure I was once falling victim to in every way possible, they had now become my life-line and provided me with the healing care I needed in my own space, my own time and my own energy without being pushed back into society to fill some societal standards or otherwise and learn how to cope with living with mental illness and finding tools to assist myself daily to return to health and well-being slowly and surely. However it was not easy by any means, it was daily struggle and immense challenges and anyone that tells you to simply snap out of it and get your shit together, simply have no idea of the battle you are fighting inside, a part of you wants to fight for your life and another part of you wants to end it all and give up and this combat between your inner victim and inner warrior is never ending, until you come out the other side. For some the warrior will be stronger and for others the victim will be stronger and this book is written for both.

As a means to inspire both the warrior and the victim inside you to never give up and seek the solutions I found for myself as well as keep looking for the solutions that show themselves to you, as we are not all the same, but when it comes to body chemistry and hormonal health, we are all built up of the same compounds and the same chemicals from the doctor may not be given to us, but the same medicine from nature is what is needed for the balance to be restored as we become what we eat and unless we move our bodies and exercise, we get imbalanced and sick and we enter our own private hell.

COMING TO TERMS WITH MENTAL ILLNESS

I decided I was going to surrender to this hell and make it my own, so I did, I made it beautiful in my surroundings, I became my own best friend and started leading a sober life, with no medication, no weed and only alcohol on rare occasions. A few years went by and all of a sudden the judicial system wrote me, they had messed up my papers and I was forced to go back and serve my time again, fortunately I was still too sick to serve my time in prison and once more were directed to the mental ward to serve my time. This time it would prove to be more beneficial than the last and I served it with greater ease and learned even more valuable aids and tools to assist myself through this process I was in, I was getting healthier by the week fast and kept working out and growing in strength and my hormone levels rapidly increasing. Eventually I was free, but after many new diagnosis and new guinea pig trials for new experimental medication I was given a shopping bag full of medication for about a month's supply, something both me and my mother found increasingly alarming and my condition would only grow worse and worse. One day when walking my dog Zorro, I decided to stop taking them all, except for the anti-psychotic one I was given for my schizoid personality disorder symptoms, something I later have come to understand as a shamanic awakening and being able to tap into people's thoughts, feelings, intent and energy were simply natural abilities for a growing empath like myself.

Upon deciding to quit cold turkey on all the others, I quickly started feeling better, the crutch of the anti-psychotic medication was just enough for me to bounce back much faster than I ever had before and I could ween myself slowly off that one as well. Eating right, more vegetables than ever and making sure I had good mineral levels and exercise every day, I started coming back to life and getting my hair back, my mind control back and eventually my complete over-all health was starting to be better than it had in decades, I was returning to full force slowly and surely.

Within 3 month's time I had regained control over my mind enough to not need the medication at all anymore and I could come more and more out of my protective bubble and start living more as I had been missing, but to full of symptoms to be able to do. Life had been missing me as much as I had been missing it and I started pushing myself. During my psychosis I had grown a tendency of using triggers as a means to prune my mind and make myself stronger, songs that would "speak to me" and things that seemed like signs from the universe were daily tools to make stronger and what was once my psychotic torment quickly became a power and force I could use to push myself mentally and emotionally. The curse had now become a gift and was growing in its giving to me daily and increasing my capacity to withstand triggers better. To call this exponential therapy would be an understatement, to call it self-torture would be more fitting, but it was just what I needed and would prove to be way more beneficial to me than any medication I ever had from the so called health industry.

The year was now 2011 and I had spent 10 years in deep depression which of 6 of those years in severe mental illness alongside severe medical mistreatment and complete isolation most of the time due to such heavy symptoms and in the end, I had nothing but my family and my beautiful and equally traumatized german shepard to lean on.

But I had become so confident through my own pruning and exposure to triggers I decided to enter social media, shortly after which I came in contact with an old flame who after a few dates became my girlfriend, we lived together for a 6 months in my tiny studio before we decided to get an apartment together, something that would lead me to relapse into alcohol, pills, weed and occasional hard substances again. This lead to a pivotal evening where we had a fight and she ended up being towed away by police.

Fortunately my land lord had heard it all and my mom's boyfriend called the police. I entered a new dark night, with massive heart openings after massive heart breaks and a short time of drug and alcohol abuse a couple of weeks on my own. I hit rock bottom once again and got myself up, I did not want to risk everything I had grown out of, to the same bad decisions and coping mechanisms that had gotten me there in the first place. So got my shit together once again and started investing further in my own health. This was when I found a wonderful herbalist online by the name of Owen Fox, who was to become a major inspiration to start eating more fruit and vegetables than I ever had before. I stopped eating meat and started eating as much living foods as I possibly could. Minimizing dairy and bread and exercising as much as possible with my 4-legged friend again. I quickly regained health and well-being and started changing my lifestyle in ways I had only dreamed about previously. I started noticing more life force pour out of me and my spiritual experience of life exponentially shifting.

I had been living with agoraphobia for so long I never thought I would have a girlfriend, let alone travel the world,

But I met a girl online who happened to live in the U.S. and the only way I was ever going to even meet her and find out if what I felt was real, was to get on a plane and go see her.

I had not even set foot on an airplane since my grandmother died when I was about 10-11 due to fear of flying but at this point I was so excited about having met someone who was also a musician that I was ready to rise to the occasion and hopefully get to make music with someone I loved.

A thought that both inspired me and excited me more than the fear of flying and I soon bought tickets and got on the plane to a country I had not felt like seeing since I was young and naïve, however my ideas and fear nation had now taken a backseat and since I had already died, what was now left of my life only seemed like a bonus life in some weird and cruel video game and the thought of growing and expanding fueled my artistic fire and nature and birthed wanderlust within this previously agoraphobic hermits heart, I now craved adventure,

I craved true love, connection and expansion, my awakening was picking up speed and nothing was going to stop me from leading the life I wanted, even if it could potentially kill me, as I had already died once and death was not something I feared anymore, however life was and I wanted to expose myself to the things I feared, like I had been for quite some time now. To someone doing exponential therapy for agoraphobia, travelling to another country alone, to meet someone you have only met online, without much funds, is a pretty big deal to say the least and I was about to dive in, head first.

However, things are not always how they seem and though sweet music could have been made, we were both too toxic and wounded to be able to make any sweet music together, in any way shape or form. She was a love avoidant and I was a love addict, a pattern that seems to play itself out in every relationship I have been in, as it mirrors my parents, where my dad was a love avoidant, hiding out in his tool shed fixing things and my mom a love addict, constantly trying to include him or receive his love and affection, but it was always on his terms and he was very rarely to be seen inside the house or in a family scenario. Someone who is a love avoidant is someone who shuts down their heart, does not verbalize affection, thoughts or feelings and developing intimacy with them is extremely difficult if not impossible, all depending on their level of avoidance and lack of vulnerability. Their avoidance will in turn trigger the need for love, affection, intimacy and ,vulnerability in the other to such an extent many even get suicidal which is an immense expression of the love addicts wounds. So here I was, discovering that not only had I been addicted to countless substances, I was also addicted to the most beautiful experience we can have on this planet, yet I was only ever attracted to those who feared expressing it, showing it and feeling it. Always ending up with someone who did not want to give me the love I so greatly needed and most willingly gave and expressed more than anyone they had ever met before. I wondered most of my life if there was someone out there who could even reciprocate my capacity to be attentive, loving, caring and vulnerable, but my wounds were not healed enough for me to attract someone like myself, we attract from our wounds after all, so we will keep attracting the same type of dynamic over and over until we get it and go "eureka!!!".

So let's take a closer look at what love avoidant and love addict is and how they may remedy this aweful dynamic according to Barbara Levinson
Ph.D, RN, LMFT, LSOTP,
CSAT Supervisor, CMAT, CST Diplomate

Love Addiction / Love Avoidance

Love can be a Battlefield. Declare Independence on Addiction to Love

Our media is dominated by the idea of the perfect love story. Romance novels, romantic comedy movies, teen dramas, popular music; some are quaint and cute, others emotional or even tragic. But all feature idealized love as their core plot device.

It's no surprise that many of us grow up with unrealistic expectations about love and romance that eventually lead to heartache and disappointment.

But what happens when this idea of perfect, idealized true love becomes an obsession? Can someone actually become addicted to love? The answer is yes.

For most people love and attraction are a natural part of life. Most of us can differentiate between an idealized Hollywood romance and reality. But for love addicts, love becomes a source of addictive emotional highs that distort the real nature of a relationship.

An addiction to love may not initially seem dangerous ... but it's a very serious mental and emotional affliction that interferes with a person's ability to establish healthy, genuine relationships.

As with any addictive substance, those addicted to love can become paranoid, and defensive and even experience symptoms of withdrawal.

Love addicts have highly unrealistic romantic expectations that put unfair pressure on their partners. They are terrified of being abandoned and will do anything to prevent it.

Many love addicts experienced a lack of nurturing and love during childhood.

Literally starved for the nurturing they didn't receive as children, they search to fill the emptiness left by their parents' neglect. For them, even a highly abusive relationship is better than being alone.

When a child's emotional needs are neglected they feel unwanted and unloved. This establishes a powerful lie in the child's mind that can eventually lead to becoming dependent on love.

They feel they're unworthy of being loved, and the only way to make the pain go away is to find someone who will give them all of the attention they were denied as children.

This kind of expectation places impossible responsibility on the partner of a love addict.

Realizing that their emotional pain and feelings of worthlessness don't go away with their partner's affections, but still terrified of being abandoned, the love addict can become resentful of their partner.

The early days of a love addict's relationships are euphoric and happy. The addicted person feels like they have met their true love, that they are destined to be with them. The fantasy creates a surge of endorphins—a literal high from love.

But as the relationship progresses, the idealized romantic dream becomes a nightmare. Coming down from their high, they become emotionally needy, clinging to their partner. Overwhelmed by the responsibility and pressure placed on them, the love addict's partner begins separating themselves from the relationship.

Unable to accept reality, the love addict holds onto fantasy for as long as possible, unwilling to face the fact that their partner is moving away from them.

When the truth finally becomes impossible to ignore, they'll begin a downward spiral of emotions. Feelings of hopelessness, abandonment, depression and panic are common.

Tormented by loneliness, the abandoned love addict will seek a new partner to heal their emotional wounds, thus beginning the cycle again.

The need to be loved at all costs is a serious mental condition that begins in childhood when you're denied the nurturing, support and affection of a loving family. If left untreated, this addiction can have the same devastating effects as chemical dependency, alcoholism or sexual addiction.

Love addiction is often connected with co-dependency, sexual addiction and abusive relationships, as well as various mental and emotional illnesses.

If you feel you're plagued by fears of abandonment, difficulty functioning without a romantic partner, and repeatedly resorting to desperate measures in order to ensure that your partner does not leave you, you can experience relief by talking with a professional therapist.

Don't despair. There are treatment options available which can help you to recognize the experiences which caused your addiction to develop... and help you learn to cope with your loneliness and heartache.

You're not alone. Don't try to resolve your heartache alone.

Love Avoidance: Conquer Your Fear of Intimacy and be Fulfilled

Are you afraid to love and be loved? Do you feel overwhelmed by your partner's emotional needs, and find yourself turning to things like work, alcohol, pornography, or infidelity to detach yourself from them?

Or maybe you feel smothered by your partners attention, wishing for more time alone, feeling obligated to give the time you give, and eager to find solace afterward?

Many musicians have built their careers on expressing the hurt and pain they've received from love lost or rejected.

Shakespeare's tragic plays reveal the sinister side of love gone wrong: jealousy, emotional torment, murder, and death.

And yet we all strive for the very thing which often brings us so much pain. The chance to find genuine connection with others, be it friendship, romance or the bond between a parent and child. We hunger for these connections and yearn to achieve them.

But for some, the pain is too much to bear. When fear of rejection, betrayal and loss overshadows the possibility of the happiness and joy that love can bring, you may find yourself desperate to avoid intimate relationships.

Love avoidants are often people who have suffered great losses and pain in their lives. Terrified of experiencing the same emotional trauma again, they take great measures to detach themselves emotionally from others.

If you are love avoidant, you might not actively avoid love itself. Love avoidants do form relationships, but are unable to allow themselves to be vulnerable with their partners. The love avoidant person is often unconscious of this behavior.

Fearful of becoming too attached or vulnerable, a love avoidant may balk at the thought of commitment, leading them to run when they start getting too close to another person.

If they manage to stay in a relationship, they may feel that something is not right or lacking, and be filled with a sense of resentment towards their partner, when their own resistance to intimacy is a major problem.

The partner of someone who is love avoidant may be at a loss to understand why their mate is becoming emotionally distant...and this often leads to conflict.

While the love avoidant may form addictions as they try to keep themselves detached—work, substance abuse, sexual affairs etc—their spouse might have no idea what triggered this behavior and begin to blame themselves.

Love avoidants often inexplicably attract love addicts. Initially the relationship may work, with the love addict showering attention and love on the love avoidant, causing them to feel accepted and cared for.

As the love addict begins bonding themselves to their partner, clinging to them for support, the love avoidant partner will inevitably begin distancing themselves, walling off their emotions from their partner.

While love addicts require constant emotional reassurance and attention as proof of a loving relationship, the love avoidant person often feels that their love is proven simply by supporting their partner on an economic and physical level.

For the emotionally avoidant person, love becomes an obligation. When their partner expresses distress over the lack of emotional intimacy in the relationship, a love avoidant person may become overwhelmed, turning to pornography, substance abuse, or workaholism as a distraction from their frustration. If it is difficult for you to be emotionally intimate with other people, if you are terrified of commitment, or feel smothered ... or love your partner but find yourself compulsively drawing away from them and seeking distraction, you may be love avoidant.

The origin of this behavior is often rooted in traumatic childhood experiences which caused significant emotional damage to the individual. Almost always the cycle of avoidance can be traced back to a destructive relationship with a parent. Through our program, you can learn to recognize how your early relationships hurt you, making it difficult to trust people and become emotionally bonded with loved ones in your adult life.

By realizing how the pattern of avoidance began, you can put a stop to the destructive cycle that has robbed you of fulfillment. You really can become vulnerable, receptive, and responsive, and enjoy the benefits of a trusting and lasting love relationship.

Definitions of Love addict and Love avoidant from Barbara's website: www.centerforhealthysexuality.com

So this was the unhealthy dynamics of every relationship I have ever had and getting into a relationship before this wound is healed is something I would advice against, as in my case I ended up married to someone who lives in another country, struggling to even file for divorce from a very toxic marriage and even though it provided me with many much needed lessons, I still could have prevented living it out to such an extent had I known and gotten help sooner. All my addictions and issues in life has been due to my unhealed childhood wounds and traumas and seeking help for these as soon as possible will only prove to serve you and prevent you from experiencing toxic and traumatic relationships and situations in life.

To assist in the cultivation your partner's intuition would be the opposite of narcissism. In my previous soul connection I was experiencing something I always missed in every relationship, backing up one another's intuitive abilities, instead of the usual relationship dynamics. As none of us were afraid to point out to the other what we saw, felt and heard with our heightening claircognizant abilities regarding one another's friends, family, snakes and sheep in wolf clothing, we had basically eliminated all reasons for "insecurity" within our partnership.

We didn't care how close you were or had been to either of us in the past, as nobody and nothing mattered more to us than our union and everything we wanted came out of our energy exchange or our unified field, anyone who were not 100% supportive were removed and anyone who made any one of our spidey senses tingle were under observation. We'd been right every time…If you made just one of us feel weird, we would talk about it and why it made us feel off and weird and strengthen and bond even stronger where most would fall short due to lack of authenticity and transparency. Something that has made us both trust one another deeper and deeper, every time the other was right, we came deeper in our trust together and placed less and less trust where it is not 100%.

We had both been disappointed by people in our blind spots the other was able to see clear as day and what would have tore down a regular relationship dynamic seemed to not work on our connection, so nothing really surprised any of us anymore, we had our tentacles out for ourselves and one another, as our connection was the most important thing to us.

We have since broken up due to many personal, health and financial issues, but remain on good terms to this writing day.

I can only speak for myself, but due to knowing human nature quite well, there is no friend I ever had I could not easily let go off, as when I was sick I was left to my own devices and "close friends" and people even made rumors- spells- black magick, saying I was dying or dead.

My INFJ - Aquarian personality has no problem sacrificing anyone or anything for the greater good so that is said.

I am not afraid to be alone anymore and that is my superpower.

I am not afraid to lose what belongs to me.

I know someone who truly loves you, cannot be taken away.

And most of all I know, if they can be easily taken,

it is not a loss, but a gain.

And I know I am a person of such value, inner and outer beauty, I would never have to be alone, this has given me an unwavering comfort in who I am and in this lack of fear of ever being alone ever again, has made my love and my force become stronger than ever and growing stronger still.

My heart, my force, my intent and my will is that of a mature, spiritual warrior and for that I am very grateful.

I am home in me, in the world, on the planet and with those who come for my work, my heart and my love.

And I will defend my home with my transparent heart and those who cannot meet me together in transparency fully, are not welcome in my home, in my space, in my circle of trust, as transparency and authentic expression is required for a harmonious life.

Trust is earned and not a given.

Trust takes years to build, seconds to break, and forever to repair.

If you want to truly go deep within a connection or union, then don't be afraid to lose one another if you speak your truth.

Truth will be recognized by those who embody it and if you speak your truth and it is not heard or felt,

you will know your partner does not stand in their own truth,

they have yet to embody their truth.

They will have a willingness to taste your truth,

without triggers, without drama, they will hear you out.

The same it is for our shadows, if someone does not have room for your shadows, they do not know their own.

There is more than enough space for all you are,

if people have space for all of themselves.

And in these spaces a true sacred union will dance in their own light, with the shadows dancing on the wall instead of within their hearts.

Learn to smell intent.

The intent will always supersede the intention, much like lucidity supersedes clarity.

With fearless transparency and lucidity our intent becomes stronger, more concise and our intuition can easier pick up other people's true intent and intention.

The intention can be wage, which is why it is harder to spot,

an intention can often be masked or hidden easily behind words and actions, while the intent is strong and you can

FEEL IT IN their words and actions.

This is why a warrior never trusts a word, but instead looks for patterns,

words are hard to trust, patterns always reveal themselves.

If we can learn to trust one another, our own selves and senses,

we no longer become less self and senseless which is what unconsciousness truly is and we don't really need to trust others, if we can fully trust ourselves. Shedding the unconscious means cultivating your senses, honing our abilities and purifying our energies so we can recognize impurities that enter our unified field. We are coming to our senses it is often said, this describes coming back to consciousness after a momentary lapse of reason and consciousness quite well.

I can smell someone's true intentions and always did from their intent they put forward in terms of energy,

this is how I stayed alive in the environment I was in for so long, I always followed my intuition as when I didn't, I got reprimanded with a lesson from higher self.

I never really needed to trust anyone, if I could trust my own senses, the more I did, the higher I went in my vibration.

Everything is learning, there are no curses upon you, only unconsciousness and that which hides there from your bloodlines many years of accumulating dysfunctional templates, patterns and programs.

But fear not,

Awareness turns a curse to a blessing as you are able to retrieve the lessons.

Wolf Medicine and Hawk Medicine is in my very name.

Wolf smells everything. Hawk sees everything.

Hawk guides Wolf to prey and away from danger.

Wolf hunts prey and protects Hawk.

Together they roam the forest in symbiosis.

So many do not receive truth from their partner as they do not give out truth to their partners.

Remember, all that is not truth comes to the surface in the light of love as love and truth are also in union.

Truth is love and Love is truth.

Deception, games, lies and agendas are all tools of untruth and not love. Know your love and know your own truth and you will recognize the lack of love in the face of untruth and the lack of truth in the face of non-love or conditional love if you will. Conditional love means I love you because this and that, it never loves for no reason, it loves with an agenda and most of us knows only this love, even from our parents, as we often felt unloved when we did something wrong.

 If you expect your partner to lie to you, you are co-creating an outcome of just that, if you expect your partner to cheat on you, you are co-creating just that, it is always co-creation,

whether we like to admit it or not, our fears also create these connections, it is either conscious or unconscious co-creation, of our friendships, our family dynamics and last but certainly not least, our relationships and sacred connections.

Bad expectations is a poor use of the imaginative faculty and co-creative abilities. Same goes with fears.

You can never expect to get anything you are not giving.

So if you fear your partner doing anything, you will be proven right in your belief if the fear is not cleared.

I have co-created a worst case scenario with soul connections, where both of our fears were produced in one another, this is usually why these connections end,

Fear of standing in true self. Fear of authenticity and transparency. Fear of love and abandonment.

Fears accumulated through the bloodline, through programs and patterns, but also through our experience of trauma in life.

Address the fears together, be willing to state your fears, this takes the fear out of your body and gives it back to the world,

so many grasp at their fears like it's a lucky straw, hoping that they will be loved and fearing that they will not, hope is an illusion, it is not real, not here yet and often makes people passive in their quest for liberation, accompanied by the fear of eventually not being loved for a truth revealed, this fear grows and festers like a cancer attaching itself to the walls of your unified field, the third energy you both are creating and soon it spreads out into your entire union, the same way the love and radiance spread out into your entire union and even bloodline.

How can you remove the fear? You can't.

Fear is energy and comes and goes.

Other people can bring fear into your field.

Be mindful and courageous.

You will have to find courage to lose everything you stand to gain, in the face of courage and honor, fears have a way of dissolving on their own and anything that can be shared and bonded on in the union will come to serve you both as one, nature and the universe favors the brave.

The merging of you two only happens in loving truth and it is gradual, over time, level by level, integrating bit by bit as you reveal more layers of your true self in your bonding.

The energy you both cultivate and spend, together and individually becomes one, one unified field of source creative energy and life force. If one of you should choose not to take care of yourself, the other will decline in health as well.

The radiance will soon diminish unless both feed their light body, exercise and take good care of mind, body and spirit.

This is a holistic connection after all and you both come together as one, to create unity and a unified field of co-creative potential and consciousness expansion.

This is not the ascension process on an individual scale,

only on a collective scale are we ascending and on an individual level we are actually descending.

Descending the higher self, into our physical vessels, this means we raise our vibrations so that higher self and those higher frequencies are possible to be cultivated and contained by and with our physical bodies, etheric bodies and so on.

Nobody is going anywhere, not into another dimension or otherwise, the fifth dimension is already here, it's a level of awareness, a rise in consciousness and frequency,

it is not far away from you and you only have to close your eyes to get there and tune into your heart, then bring it with you in your daily life.

 Any other ideas of the fifth dimension being a "there" is fabricated mumbo-jumbo from the new age indoctrination machine which is a corrupt money making organ like any other.

To become free, we have to look at our ideas, ideologies, belief systems, to see how we are keeping ourselves locked.

Remember ANYTHING is a belief system.

Even astrology and human design, twin flames and simpler smaller human beliefs, even if these tools work and we can use them to improve our lives, they are still based in a belief as belief is initial to experience often handed to us or stolen during childhood and teenage years and deeply engrained in us, such as religion and so on. And most anything defined with earthly eyes has another definition beyond this planet. If you can understand this, you will come far in navigating your earthen experience. If not, you will come to struggle in your awakening process. And you can consciously use these systems to create reality. Any belief you will be proven right about if there is enough energy behind it. Once you realize this, your magick will become very powerful.

"Magick is the bloodstream of the universe, forget what you know, or think you know. All that you require is your intuition."
- Willow

PHYSICAL MOVEMENT TO SHIFT MENTAL IMBALANCE

The main key apart from God's pharmacy and mindfulness practices such as meditation and observing one's own mind in my humble opinion is movement. Moving the lymphatic waste and sweating out toxins is a sure way to boost your hormone levels and assist your mind, body and spirit to heal itself.

Your body has the capacity to heal anything if you create the environment it needs in order to heal.

So how do we create an environment for the body in order for it to heal? First and foremost we must eliminate toxins from our intake, preferably completely, but minimizing intake to a low minimum while increasing healthy intake and increasing exercise will of course yield results, but complete elimination of toxins as well as a deep detox will give the best results in my own personal experience.

Apart from moving the lymphatic system through movement, hormones are also increased and balanced through exercise and will leave a mentally instable person feeling improvement of mental faculty fairly quickly.
And if you really want to boost the endocrine system and lymphatic system I highly suggest herbs to further speed along your healing and yield the most optimal results at fast pace.
Herbs like Schizandra berries, Maca, Ashwagandha and other adaptogenic herbs offer an amazing healing property to you, as the herbs adapt to your own healing needs, in other words it will balance out your hormones whether you have too high or too low levels the adaptogens serve you in such a way you are left balanced either way. The schizandra berry being a five flavor berry, it works on all the 5 major organs, it works on all the 5 energy bodies and all the 5 physical senses.
It is also a major sexual tonic which increases libido, vigor and fertility which are good signs of life force having increased.

Nature heals, we already know that, we have known that for thousands of years and only until recently given up all our sovereignty and accountability for our own health and well-being to our local physicians and allopathic medicine practitioners. But we used to be more sovereign as natural healers until the last few centuries in decreasing numbers on a vast scale. But most of us in the western culture, hail from druid and shamanic ancestry where natural medicine was at the center of folk-lore and part of the healing traditions from generation to generation. This is the way of the dream of Gaia, the natural dream we as dream weavers are meant to weave, The original dream of harmony and health for all of mankind.

As I have mentioned earlier in the book, physical movement is alpha omega and adding good, rich nutrition to your body to build cells and regenerate your mind and body is vital to your healing. Nothing comes without a price and the price of true and lasting healing is to change your lifestyle.
Diets never worked for me and it doesn't seem to work for most people, at least not when it comes to lasting health.
Only a lifestyle change that supports your regeneration 100% instead of producing decay like processed foods and lack of accountability for what goes into the body, will without a doubt produce results. I have seen it time and time again, those that wishes for their healer to wave a magical wand for them to be alright and not put in any effort themselves, always revert back to their health problems through an endless loop of quick fix schemes or allopathic trials without changing their lifestyle, Never get the results they want, especially not long-term.
So as I tell my clients, I can only help you as much as you are willing to help yourself. First and foremost, you are the obstacle standing in your own way of true and lasting health.
What you put in your body, how well you take care of your body and genetics play a major role in your healing.
But what if I told you, that DNA and genetics can be altered? Healed?

What most people see as hereditary and bad ancestral genetics, are in fact patterns, programs and templates, that can be altered on an etheric level into the physical as everything starts in energy. The things that were handed down through your bloodlines are to be found in your etheric body, mental body, pain body, emotional body and then the physical body.

You are the result of your parents lack of love for themselves, meaning their poor lifestyle choices and living in decay prior to your conception is what made up their cells and which was also the foundation for your early body make-up.

If your parents had poor lifestyles (like most of our parents in this day and age) your cells and everything you physically are, is made up of the fabrics from their lifestyle choices, but every 7 years our bodies are completely rearranged and changed and so we can turn this around for ourselves once we become accountable for our own mind, body and spirit. So in the end, nobody is to blame but ourselves if we are not well, living well and taking care of our body.

We can alter our bodies, we can heal our genetics and yes, we can optimize our own physical health through etheric work, through mindfulness and living from the heart.

Heart centered consciousness heals not only ourselves and our lives, but it spreads into other people's lives around us and most importantly our respective bloodlines.

This is part of the work for many who have incarnated onto planet earth in this time, to heal the dysfunctional links in the chain for their ancestral bloodline and this setting the children of tomorrow free from their ancestral dispositions,

Which are many for the many.

Not only can we think ourselves healthy with a good mindset and understandings of metaphysical reality, but we can take actions physically as well to make sure our body is manifested from sparkly living cells that thrive and glow of electricity.

That is what you are, an electric being in an electric universe and your charge and your power stems from the frequency and charge of the food you eat. We literally do become that which we eat, that which we think of, align ourselves with, the abyss eventually looks back on the observer, so it is very important to keep a healthy mind about and be mindful of your thoughts, when you cannot rearrange them or clear your mind, go for

walks, work out, play with your pet, watch a movie with a loved one or by yourself and to have better control of your own mind, meditation and exercise are the two greatest tools alongside nutrition that can heal a mental imbalance completely.
I quit medication from the doctors and 3 months after with my healing regime I was free of symptoms to an adequate and promising level to keep going where I was going.
I so quickly felt better and did better it was no question for me what had been the worst culprit to my imbalances,
The experimental and new and improved medicines of the allopath mental health club. They were playing Russian roulette with my life, well-being and mental health on the line,
Reduced to a simple guinea pig for the medical community to fiest on and experiment with in order to show promising results on me, with their particular solution for my ailments.
In the end, I had not much faith left in the western medicine, "one pill had made me larger and the other made me small", 5 medicines and 3 pills for the severe side effects of the other 5 and a sleeping pill. Most all of which were psychotropic in nature, yet with no noticeable stimulant effect other than a fried brain, restless leg syndrome, skin rash and itching and occasional jolts inside your brain from neuro rewiring.
Whatever they were, they were not medicinal in any way, they were clearly lobotomizing me with legal chemicals in order to make me a more reliable citizen, more dosile, more sheep-like,
After all they had tons of experience and a PHD, how were they not to be trusted? And most of all, how can health not be their field of expertise when they are trained physicians...
No, I am really asking, look it up, nutrition and balance of the body is not something they teach in you in "medical school".
That is something you will have to research and realize for yourselves if you haven't already, most of our social constructs and organizations are corrupt to the core and dissected so that there can be no good communication across the boards.
We have one doctor for every part of the body, yet we cannot have our body treated as a whole, holistically?
Something so absurd and surrealistic could only be an excerpt from a children's book, could it really be so?
The world we live in is a crazy one, we already established that

earlier in the book if you hadn't already.

So your best bet is to learn how to be your own doctor if you are to come out of this with your life intact, otherwise pills with suicidal tendencies as a side-effect will be your trajectory until the day you die most likely. Something I am trying to prevent with this book you are holding in your hand.

And I hope you pass it on to your friends, so they also may benefit from its content and become accountable for their own health and wellbeing, nothing like becoming sovereign to any being, to master one's own self and reality.

When I first decided to quit my medication and start eating right and moving my body more, I had no idea how long it would take to heal myself, as I at the time was still under the belief that traditional household foods were enough to heal my body, something that could not be further from the truth.

It is now September 2017 as I am writing this and as I started writing the book until now, I have quit smoking, started running, quit processed foods, cheese, milk, meat and everything that has been sabotaging my healing the past decade. You see, dairy products and processed chemical food like products are two of our most toxic components to our healing that gives us stagnant lymphatic fluids and messes up our endocrine system fundamentally which in turn keeps our bodies from fully healing. So both I have now gone full on raw in the time of writing this, now even cooked foods as they slow down our detox, only raw living foods that assist the body in moving the lymphatic waste, herbs that boost the endocrine and a good healthy lifestyle with lots of exercise.

I never liked running, I would not run unless I was being chased or was chasing the bus, it just never appealed to me, A program of it not being cool or feeling good in my teen years, as I also had asthma growing up, physical activity like that was hard on my body and lungs. But as spiritual accountability increases and I more and more realize what it takes to truly heal and not just hope to heal, but take full measures in order to transcend my illness and traumas in life, doing things that are naturally good for my body and making better decisions for myself and my partner seems to come a lot more easily.

When we know better, we do better, it is that simple, which is why I wish to inform the world that most of the imbalances we see today, even mental imbalance, has a lot to do with nutrition and lifestyle more than anything else. A condition can reversed with the right knowledge and actions, as I am living proof of. So I went along and bought running shoes about a year ago and started interval training to boost my levels rapidly, however I was still smoking cigarettes which was holding my healing back substantially. But the more I ran the better I felt and the easier it was to let go off the cigarettes and invest full time in cultivating this amazing feeling of increasing health and well-being. I used to believe that if the amount of good things you did for your body outweighed the bad things, you were still on the right track, but for a decade this would prove to keep my healing process at a very slow pace, only once I removed all toxins and stopped adding bad things to my body did I truly start detoxing and healing at a rapid rate.

So make the choice today, what can you do on a daily basis to start helping you grow in the right direction, start small like I did, but maybe at a faster pace if you'd like fast results, I only wish I had known a decade ago what I know now.

Make yourself the daily healing agenda, where you list what you are going to do for your mind, body and spirit in order to heal, what you are going to eat and what you are going to do of exercise, maybe healing modalities, meditations or other things that will prove to help you heal from years of toxic living.

Keep a healing journal, write down post-its with inspirational cues to your own healing or other things you can think of that can help keep you on track towards your complete holistic healing. Whatever you choose in the beginning, make sure you don't bite over too much, you don't want to lose inspiration and hopes of achieving what you would like, so set small goals that are manageable and realistic or you will only sabotage your own efforts and give up. Make it fun and most of all, push yourself a little every day, whether it be a fear, an obstacle or anything else. You can do whatever you put your mind to and I am living proof of that and if I can, so can you. All it takes is will power and determination and being sick of being sick, which you most likely are since you are holding this book in your hand.

Movement is alpha omega to healing and in the beginning I started out walking 30 mins a day, then an hour and eventually now I am running an hour a day, something that seemed very unlikely to me only a couple of years ago. But I have to fight in order to stay here, it is a daily struggle to inspire, motivate and follow through and maintain optimal health, sometimes I end up one step ahead and two steps back and I would be lying if I said it is easy, it is in no way easy. The only way to keep it fun for me, if I go at it with the warrior spirit, see my health and well being as the battle field and to come out the victor of my challenges. It helps me to stay focused as a warrior and not let my guard down for too long over time, as it reminds me of where I am being attacked from all angles at all times and to stay alert with the challenges I am facing on a daily basis.

I cannot stress the importance of a daily healing agenda enough, so I will mention it again, create a regime for yourself where you apply yourself a little or a lot every day to your own healing and increase and adjust according to energy, needs and timeframe and you will eventually find yourself in a place of healing and see such results you will not want to go back to your old ways of decay and decline. Stalking death means cultivating vitality and life force and stalking the very things that keep you in decay and decline and minimizing them in your life. I have since started writing this book actually found a healthier mindset when it comes to healing and that is to also occasionally allow myself to enjoy some toxins and have a good time as well, to have balance in life, but in the beginning I recommend eliminating toxins and decaying foods and lifestyle all together in order to heal deeper and more thorough, but as you start seeing the results you work hard for, you should allow yourself to enjoy certain things here and there without beating yourself up like I did, only causing you to want more comfort foods for being so hard on yourself and eventually leading to a slippery slope of comforting yourself for being hard on yourself. The mind will trick us any way it can in order to sabotage our efforts and keep us the way we were as ego fears change more than anything and will sneak in the backdoor and talk us into our old ways when we aren't even looking.

THE LONG WAY BACK TO HEALING

The road to healing is filled with distractions, setbacks and dangers and the greatest of these is allopathic medicine, for the very reason that you have to heal twice from the same ailments, once from what you truly ailed and second from the medication prescribed by your doctors, most of which is highly toxic with side-effects that makes any condition worse than it was initially before starting traditional western allopathic treatment.

Another one would be the many alternative modalities out there in which some are very outdated, but the main reason why people remain stagnant in their healing, I as a holistic healer see, is the fact that we expect results too fast and go for quick fixes and from modality to modality in order to find the magic wand, whereas if we stuck with one modality long enough so we'd find what truly works through a process of trial and error. But people want the quick fix and that is why they would rather pop a pill than change their lifestyle, but in the long run this is something that is not working to their benefit, something we see on the rise in today's society, more and more people are getting really sick and more and more people are trying alternative ways of finding health.

I can tell you right here and right now that there is no quick fix to whatever it is you are battling, only long term investment in your own health is going to save you and you yourself have to learn how to become your very own best friend and take actions on a daily basis in order to truly heal yourself, there is no way around that. You can go to healer after healer and try modality after modality, but unless you invest in your own healing, you will most likely not see the results you wish to see and if you do, it most likely will not last, unless you put in time and effort and create a daily healing agenda for yourself.

The more healthy choices you do for yourself , the more you will heal and get lasting results, the most healthy choice you can do is completely eliminate toxins, eliminate one toxin at a time, start with the easiest one so you get inspired and motivated to keep letting go off toxins in your life, the problem is most of what people call food on this planet, is in fact toxins. And food addiction is by far the hardest addiction I personally have had to face and quit, because food-like products are everywhere and everyone is eating it, serving it and you have to be firm and decisive and stay strict with yourself.

Dr. Robert Morse is one of my greatest mentor's when it comes to detox and true health and after trying many things for my candida and parasites, trial and error, I landed on Dr. Morse's raw fruitarian and herbal regimes and having faster results than I ever had eating even something as nutritious as organic cooked vegetables, my body simply didn't detox enough for us to see the results I wanted to see. Within a few days of doing a parasite cleanse I had flukes and parasites coming out of me and 8 out of 10 are filled to the rim with parasites and most people on a classic traditional diet have candida and even acidosis. Acidosis will eventually lead to cancer, so you see why we have such a health crisis on this planet in our day and age, it all boils down to nutrition.

Same for mental illness, the brain needs the minerals to work and the hormones in balance, in order to function optimally.

So we will look at how you can balance the mind in some easy to follow steps:

First of all I will say that supplementation has little to no use for you as you will most likely not take up what your body needs.

So if you want to add minerals to your body, you will have to get them from a nutrient dense and rich plant diet, lettuce, leafy greens, superfoods are my personal go-to's for balanced intake of minerals.

Then add the herbs mentioned earlier and move the herbs in your body around with physical activity of your choice for them to get to all the corners and cells in your body.

This way you regenerate cells and boost your hormone levels, This is the fastest way to heal yourself I have found in my decades in search of the optimal healing regime.

Coffee Enemas and liver flushes, kidney flushes etc are the alpha and omega for healing as you remove so much waste and toxins and built up toxins in the organs, stones in the kidneys, gallbladder and not to mention the mucoid plaque in the intestines, as a result the absorption of nutrients magnifies substantially.

Vitamins I get in plentiful from the fruits, Here I also eat for my needs, bananas and oranges as much as possible, at least an apple and an avocado a day, pineapples and mangosteen, kiwi's and the occasional papaya, passionfruit or dragonfruit, but watermelon is my personal favorite superfood for so many reasons and moving the lymphatic is one of my favorite uses of watermelon and my most favorite fruit to get loads of nutrients and move the lymphatic system and detox at the same time as boosting my body with delicious frequencies, I can assure you, within a short period of time you will feel the difference. Watermelon fasts are highly detoxing as well as super boosting and I highly recommend mono-diets of watermelon and astringent fruits as Dr. Morse says, with only fruit I saw healing take place I had long waited to see and I only wish I had known when I began what I know now as I could have cut my healing time down several years with the knowledge I have of the endocrine and lymphatic system at this time in my life. Detoxing and balancing these will prove to optimize health, performance, quality of life and over-all change everything in your life as it will make you more energized, well rounded off individual, more balanced in mind, body and spirit.

Our environment contains endless copious amounts of toxins, trace metals and radiation and the only way to combat a constant decay of our mind, body and spirit, detoxing as well as boosting our system is of utmost importance.
With the increase of radiation in our climate from the Fukushima crisis the mainstream media has apparently gently swept under the rug, we now see ocean life and sea food being highly affected by the exposure to radiation already and with what they are spraying the skies with as well, we are being bombarded with toxins on a daily basis.

Iodine supplementation is one supplementation we should not be without, eating lots of kelp and algae like Chlorella and Spirulina is very good for heavy metal detoxing and radiation exposure. Apart from what is in our environment we also have chemicals we wash our houses with, chemicals on our clothes, bed sheets, everywhere there are chemicals right down to the things we put in our bodies, food-like products and synthetic medicine artificially derived many times from the very herbs and plants we so-called alternative health practitioners use to treat the very same illness, but with half the healing time and none of the side effects that these synthesized drugs produce. They seek to synthesize everything so that they can patent it and make money from our illness, rather than actually treat an illness as there is simply no business in a healthy population. We see a financial interest in our healing with such ramifications on our entire societal structure that entire generations are facing a major health crisis, not to mention mental health crisis as a result of these big companies playing Russian roulette with the collective mental health of the people of planet earth. I don't think the institutions and the health system are prepared for an increasingly vast number of spiritual awakenings and the collective mental health crisis they are facing, least of all equipped, unless we count their medical approach which is laughable at best. We need spiritually equipped and experienced people to guide the collective when the shit hits the fan with everything that is no longer working, evolution always finds a way and we are in dire need of evolution as a people, as a species and as individuals.

We long for a better connection to ourselves, to animals, the planet and find our place in the cosmos and live out our grand design, personally and as a collective, the human design, the dream of the planet, the harmonious utopia our planet truly can become with a planet of spiritually mature and accountable beings. Spiritual accountability starts with ourselves, our own mind, body and spirit. Accountable for how we think, feel, speak, act and create our reality, down from our very health, to our interactions and creation of reality throughout our day. Accountable for how we treat others, how we let others treat us, What goes in and out of our bodies, how we care for ourselves and others and how present we are with those we are present with. Spiritual accountability is more than just what we eat, it is what we think, what we speak, don't speak, how we act and are with ourselves and one another. It is virtuous living with integrity and transparency and being the best version of yourself with the awareness that you currently possess.

As once we know better, we do better.

One of my personal favorite sayings of all time. We truly do better once we have a better understanding, we all wish to evolve and grow and become a better version of ourselves, even though we all fight resistance within and without in terms of self-sabotage, self-importance and lack of lucidity, we all have blind spots and denial working against us, so I have found adapting to the warrior spirit and a warrior mentality in terms of the ongoing spiritual warfare on my mind, body and spirit from the very existence itself, has proven to be of utmost importance. I am not only fighting an enemy without, but I have an adversary deeply programmed into me which I have to combat in order to regain my vitality. A parasitic lifeform that feeds of my disdain, misery and lack of vitality, a program placed into our entire bloodline producing lack of self-love and self-destructive tendencies and I have made it my life's mission to eradicate these programs, patterns and templates.

I want nothing more feeding of my bloodline, I want nothing to stand in the way of my bloodlines freedom to live in peace and harmony once we have cleared these things once and for all.

I am not alone in this mission anymore, my family are all well aware of the clearing work we now are doing as so much of it has surfaced to be healed the last few years and has been the most transformational work I have ever been part of within my own family structure. Finding the ancestral patterns and breaking the chains will show itself in every direction of your bloodline and you will see your grandparents as well as your children change from the energies being lifted out of the bloodline. Ancestral clearings is one of my specialties as a healer and I do this work on an etheric level so once it is cleared you will feel lighter in your energy, mood and physical body, Like a weight has been lifted and family dynamics change and sometimes I even see people's appearance change with the change of energy in the bloodline. Energy work is a necessity when it comes to healing ourselves and without it I would not be at the level of consciousness or of the health I am today, had it not been for the initiations from spirit and the training from teachers along the way to optimize my understanding of the etheric body and the cosmic alchemy of life.

My teachers have been put in my path one by one and they have all been great men in their own right, great thinkers and more so amazing feelers. Divine masculine from the previous paradigm, a bit harder and still wounded many of them,
Yet stronger teachers, more loving teachers, you'd have to search long and wide for, of this I am extremely grateful.
The universe and higher self always had a tendency to nudge me in the right directions and set up the right meetings at the right time for change to occur in my life, in my awareness.
With every new teacher, a new level of awareness was achieved every time, not always as fast as some of them would like as I am a hard learner and I lose interest fast if it is something I don't catch on to right away, something I have done in other lifetimes and perfected in my being, doing anything else simply has me lose interest and radiance and at times in life, even my will to live. My will goes hand in hand with the ability to be myself. If I can be myself and do what I am good at, what I love, I feel happy, in the flow, seen, heard, like I belong and this is why I want others to come home to blueprint as well. If we had a planet of people living from blueprint, we would most likely not have war I believe truthfully. Nobody would be willing to fight for anything but their dreams, their passions, their lovely life created by will, intent, consciousness and abundance from being in alignment with who they truly are. When we are naturally ourselves, life flows naturally for us, This is natural law, cosmic laws, if we live naturally, we will naturally have a better life, it is simple logic.

MINDFULLNESS AND MEDITATION

There are certain practices that we can make to assist our mind in healing from mental illness and one of the most important tools in the beginning for me, was mindfulness, self-healing (energy work) and most importantly meditation.

Nobody can take control of our mind for us and nothing does it so fast as being mindful and meditate, raise your awareness and become the observer of your thoughts, feelings and energy.

We produce our energy from our thoughts and feelings which in turn affects our mind, body and spirit and health. So it becomes detrimental to make an effort to understand the mind, our thoughts and why we think the things we do. Walking meditation was one of the more easier ways in which I was able to regain the control of my mind and have less imbalanced thoughts and a better filter for thoughts and unwanted thoughts and even voices. I always had a very hard time calming down enough to sit still and relax and the times I didn't, I had a hard time silencing the mind and getting distracted.

I soon came to realize that this was my ego highly in resistance to anything that might alleviate me from its clutches on how I perceive myself and the world. The damaged ego will sabotage any attempt in the beginning for the seeker to find his or her peace and every trauma and event will be thrown at you in your mind's eye until every little thing you have experienced has been processed, then and only then have I been able to find those moments of stillness that expands into the center of your

creation where you are perceiving infinity in the everlasting now. When my mind had moments of not thinking a thought, I got scared in the beginning, what if I never am to think again and you realize you have already started thinking, we are so trained to constantly yammer in our minds that not having a thought is frightening to most I have spoken with. Many don't know how to meditate and make up all these rules in their minds about how it should look, feel and be and when it doesn't instantly turn into Samadhi, many turn away, thinking they are doing it wrong or other ideas of meditation,
I know as I was one with all of the above.

I hated meditation, to spend time with my screaming silence in my mental illness, to go into those wounds, but I was forced into solitude and silence and quickly learned to love it. I had to, or I would go mad as so many had suspected I was, but I was only having a shamanic awakening and if I would have had a shamanic mentor I most likely would have kept a lot more of my psychic abilities intact, but they are now all returning, ten years after and in my balanced state now, they may be the gifts they were intended be and not the curse they were perceived as back then. While I was in the mental institution I had an amazing Mexican doctor named Omar, we often spoke of Carl Gustav Jung's dream work and shamanism and would always end our sessions in a meditation. I quickly came into my peace when I was in solitude in this way and found my strength enough to push through the horrors of my own mind, the anxiety, the paranoia, the visions and sights I would see in waking state as my paranormal senses had opened up a Pandora's box of an interdimensional reality.
I now communicated with interdimensional beings, the nature, animals, insects, everything was now speaking to me 24/7 365 days out of the year and synchronicity and mystical experiences was now an ocean I was swimming in more and more as opposed to how I was drowning psychotically in the beginning. I am just about hundred percent certain that my choice to start eating healthier at the rehab facility and get loads of sleep, meditation, cognitive therapy as well as me and Omar's brotherly talks on spirituality and his amazing therapy is what

saved me in the end, made me strong enough to sit through the mental torment I was constantly living in. Hearing and feeling people's thoughts, intentions and seeing into possible timelines and alternate realities while in a highly criminal environment is not easy for such a highly sensitive being. I was not in the right places any longer for someone with my talents, gifts or traits, if talents like these get in the wrong hands people could be killed with just thought alone and without a heart centered consciousness like mine, I am certain that people like me are used as weapons. I am not sure what they wanted with me when I was targeted and constantly stalked by a group of paramilitary individuals, but I am sure it was a fight for my life force, my light and power and they would park near my house, follow the car, pop up everywhere, the same people and once I showed absolutely no fear and that I was willing to fight to the death and take as many as possible with me if I had to, it all ended.

It was like a trial by fire, a war for my consciousness and power and they had no idea who they were up against, I had no problems even bullying my own mind and self as that is what I had been programmed to do as a child being bullied, the abuse I had experienced as a child and also given to myself in my teen years and beyond made what they could potentially do to me, harmless, as I had done far worse things to myself, by my own hand.

I was my own worst enemy and they knew it, they tried their best to make me devour myself from the inside out, but to little avail as I was a spirit not so afraid to die. I had been on the other side so many times throughout my years of psychedelic exploration and overdoses that when faced with a god-defying act I had no problems facing death and in the end, ended up making a death defying act as well.

I was shown I could not die, I was not allowed to leave yet, I had more to do and spirit was going to guide me, train me and keep me alive as long as I would listen to spirit and surrender to what it wanted me to do, I would live to see all my coal, be turned to gold it said. It has now been 10 years since my last severe suicide attempt and I am sitting here writing a book about how I indeed turned my coal to gold, this is my process consciously and unconsciously, the process has remained true to its nature and purified all aspects of mind, body and spirit sometimes gradually and sometimes instantly in a quantum leap of awareness into another plateau of understanding of the mechanics of metaphysical nature and shamanic awareness of energy, life, love and the many facets of existence throughout the multiverses.

But for the most part it has been gradual expansion and growth over a period of 10 years, with the descent being almost the same as the time it has taken to heal and integrate it all as well.

But like I have mentioned earlier, if I had truly done back then what I know now, these 10 years in healing could have easily been made into 2-3 years with the understanding of nutrition, the lymphatic and endocrine system that I have now and it baffles me that western medicine is not trained better in terms of nutrition and lifestyle as much as they are chemicals, allopathic medicine and their designated non-holistic part of the body. With a dissected understanding of a holistic being it is a downright spiritual amputation of holistic ideals and will soon come to create even more imbalances in an already imbalanced body. It is time western medicine is revised and the original, natural medicine made legalized and available to all,

So that those who choose spiritual sovereignty are free to do so without harm to anyone person, animal, group of people or otherwise. Highly ethically conscious beings should be allowed to work in the best interest of source creation and be in alignment with the original intent for the blueprint of all of creation, including our own bodies, minds and spirits. This is the future of mankind, to return to the original blueprint, so that we will live out our destiny as individuals and as a collective of humans, in order to do so, we have to remember who we are and we now have several beings on earth who remember who they are as a soul and these beings are assisting others in returning to their innocence, their hearts and passions, talents and soul gifts so that they can embody who they are as a soul and consciousness and this makes all mental illness obsolete.

If everyone did what they wanted to do and were excellent at, there would not be jealousy, greed, envy or opposing force to your creations as everyone would be too busy creating and co-creating their own and the collective dream.

My mentor and friend Mark Cloudfoot Gershon calls this dream the dream of the planet, it is the original dream of Gaia, it holds the utopia that we all could live in if we heal the timelines in question that can lead to either a possible heaven or a possible hell, all depending on humanities current efforts and consciousness involved in our evolution, pollution of resources and state of affairs.

In this dream of the planet, we are allowed in to the cosmic councils and join the galactic family of interdimensional beings throughout the multiverses, in this dream of the planet, we are living in harmony again with all that is and thriving to the best of our collective capacity and the planet and all its resources with us.

I often share Mark's material with my friends and loved ones as it is the material that has helped me understand who I am as a soul and being more than any other material I have come across on my path, even more than Carlos Castaneda and even Carl Jung, as I find the deathdefier and his unique Toltec perspective to be very similar to my own experience.

The Gateway Of Light technique he teaches is very similar to how I discovered the energy in my palms and how I would heal myself in my shamanic awakening. It creates a stronger unified field and thus increases your vitality as well, as everything starts in energy and this was the beginning of the healing of all my dis-ease, it helped me find calm with my panic attacks and it helped me prepare myself with peace when facing my agoraphobia and going to the store after months of preparing by riding to the store and waiting in the car. Moment for moment moving one step closer to my liberation, to the freedom of my own self-imposed phobias and extreme anxiety, schizophrenic thoughts in medical terms, it was not an easy task and I knew I would have to devote years to recover from the deep soul torment I was in and with the help of my family, especially my mother, I have been able to take the time to heal slowly and surely and come back to health. Anything can be healed with the right environment, compassion, empathy and understanding of the mind, body and spirit.

Understanding energy and how energy manifests illness is of utmost importance to become your own healer, without accountability of thoughts, words and actions we keep creating more illness in ourselves and others through unconscious energy and unconscious manifestation.

Black magic is practiced every day in the simple words we use, like when I hear someone say "fuck my life" or "fuck the world" or "they can go to hell", I remind them of the power of the word. Learning to control my imagination with mental imbalance has been my hardest challenge, but most rewarding as well, I still have not recovered all my spiritual gifts from the medication I was on, but they have all slowly been returning since detoxing and gradually opening myself up to the energies and using my talents, gifts and traits, has made them all slowly and surely return over time, nothing is lost, only improved.

Black magic is simply unconsciousness, programs and patterns like gossip and other popular culture related negative programming and unconsciousness, as we see that once people truly come to consciousness they have little time for such mindless unconscious destructive non-sense and I do my best to nip gossip in the butt when I hear it and you can be sure of one thing, those who gossip to you, gossip about you too, that never fails.

Keeping conscious company as much as possible has become an act of self-love as well, as people with nothing to lose and people cultivating unconsciousness is a downright hazard to creating a conscious and balanced life as these people leave a trail of misfortune, havoc and drama in their trails. And if it is one thing I have learned that my mind, body and spirit is highly allergic to it is drama and stress and unconscious people need drama like we others need oxygen and we become like the company we keep. We are basically all the people we know, the books we have read, the music we have listened to, this is how much programming affects us and how impressionable the mind is for programming, we become like the company we keep. We become like the entertainment we expose ourselves to, for good or bad. Where my focus and attention goes, my energy goes, if I put my energy and consciousness towards destruction, destruction will find its way back around into my life somehow, if I put my energy and consciousness towards creation, creation will find its way back around in my life somehow, it is a simple philosophy and has made my life so much simpler to navigate, planting seeds of creation where I go, planting seeds of consciousness where I go and gifting people a healing word, a healing thought, a healing touch wherever you go and be the peace and healing of that place. All it takes is a shift in consciousness, from worrier to warrior, from victim to warrior. Another wonderful shaman that has helped me along the way is Clay Lomakayu, medicine of one, where he talks of the victim and the warrior and the circle of one, we create a circle of healing. I highly recommend his book and you tube channel for those seeking to heal sorrow and anger or to understand someone better, who is healing these things. It lead me to better understand how a wound could express itself in two ways, it could express itself inwardly or outwardly and either make one a soft victim or a hardened warrior, but at the core, in the wound, the same futility and need for love is the very same. On the path of heart it is more difficult to develop a hardened heart as we adapt to the warrior spirit, but it is one thing to keep in mind, how the warrior may end up with a hardened heart should we not proceed with great care and thread lightly and lovingly on this path of heart.

To cause others harm and inflict pain on others because we ourselves are hurting is never ok, hurt people hurt people, but it is up to us to end the vicious cycles of abuse somehow and seek healing for ourselves and our traumas in life.

Spiritual accountability also shows us how we are affected by the way we affect other people and so eventually we change our ways as we realize how we may not have such a positive impact on the people around us acting out of wounds and reliving patterns of trauma over and over. The very definition of insanity is to do the same thing over and over expecting a different result, so it goes without saying it would drive even the best of us entirely mad to keep looping in the same family dysfunctions year after year. These patterns and programs are etheric in nature and thus energy and can be removed by an experienced etheric surgeon and energy worker. I have found in my experience, the best way to go about working on these dysfunctions and traits is both physically from the awareness of them and break them, but I have also found that working with them in the etheric sheet bodies is equally as important or the traits, patterns and programs all too quickly return upon exposure to re-templating, re-programming from peers, friends, family and society. We expose ourselves to programs, patterns, templates and consciousness every day from the moment we open our eyes to the time we go to bed and beyond as even our dreams hold implants and programs as well, we are never truly free from exposure to the matrix and it should be kept in mind at all times through our exposure we are programming ourselves with TV, music, books, people, conversations and so on and so forth and to look past the firmament of human construct as often as possible to keep our awareness and focus aligned with our blueprint and construction of our very own dream and reality, as when we are busy dreaming another's dream into reality, we have very little time for our own, something the establishment and our society is well aware of and why they seek to distract you at any given time with billboards and suggestions for trains of thought to pass through a very susceptible and unconscious consciousness. To cultivate our own consciousness and creation consciously is of course our greatest imperative to win this war for our consciousness, for our health, mind, body and spirit. To cultivate our lucidity and raise above levels of consciousness that seek to train the mind to imprison itself in worry and cancer producing mentality and keep your mind, body and spirit in a constant restless state of fight or flight until you become so imbalanced you need medication in order to cope with the reality they are feeding you, this reality construct that we have to come to know as the dream of the world, the illusion, the matrix. None of which is real to anyone but those who part-take in the sustenance and co-creation of this dream through the news, the

TV programming, the mainstream music, movies, books and the gossip, slander and collective bullying of popular cultures main characters in mainstream media.

All of which is to be found within the bubble of consciousness known as planet earth's collective consensus of reality.

Our very definitions, our very words are all earthly words, definitions and programs and hold very little meaning past the stratosphere or the firmament as many alchemists have called it throughout human history. Beyond the firmament our consciousness is formless, it is still open to mystery, to not knowing and to challenge our very definitions as our capacity for human understanding and consciousness evolves past the current consensus for what is real, possible and agreed upon as reality. In order to truly set our minds free as awakening shamans, it becomes imperative to understand that culture is not real and that everything we observe is not free from the observer, we affect everything in our holographic experience of reality from our thoughts, feelings, belief systems, patterns, programs and templating from our bloodline and country.

We come to find that everything we believed in, we stole from somebody else and made it our own somehow, somewhere along the way and we defended it tooth and nail as if it was our own, as if we were the very thing we were defending, whether it would be nationality, skin color, creed, religion, music, sports or our very new age beliefs who seem much like religion.

It does not matter what we installed ourselves with or what we choose to uninstall, we will always have belief systems and programs in order to run and operate in the matrix, our machine, our computer needs an operating system, a human one, in order to function in third dimensional reality.

8 GOD'S PHARMACY AND HERBALISM

In this chapter we will take a closer look at just how harmful western medicine pharmacopeia truly is to the chemical make-up of your body and so in turn mind and spirit and the science behind the destruction made on our physical vessels truly is and just how far this rabbit hole goes from a scientific angle presented to you from a medical and nutritional point of view.

The following excerpts are taken from the book;
Antidepressants, Antipsychotics and Stimulants
by Dr. David W. Tanton, Ph.D.

1. Adderall depletes: Vitamin B12, Vitamin C, and potassium.

2. Prozac depletes: Vitamin B1 , Vitamin B2, Vitamin B3, Vitamin B 6, Vitamin B 12, Folic Acid, Vitamin C, Vitamin D, Coenzyme Q10, Calcium, Magnesium, Manganese, Selenium, Sodium, Zinc, and Glutathione.

3. Paxil depletes: Vitamin B1, Vitamin B2, Vitamin B3, Vitamin B6, Vitamin B12, Folic Acid, Vitamin C, Vitamin D, Coenzyme Q10, Calcium, Magnesium, Manganese, Selenium, Sodium, Zinc, and Glutathione.

4. Zoloft depletes: Vitamin B1, Vitamin B2, Vitamin B3, Vitamin B6, Vitamin B12, Folic Acid, Vitamin C, Vitamin D, Coenzyme Q10, Calcium, Magnesium, Manganese, Selenium, Sodium, Zinc, and Glutathione.

5. Celexa depletes: Vitamin B1, Vitamin B2, Vitamin B3, Vitamin B6, Vitamin B12, Folic Acid, Vitamin C, Vitamin D, Coenzyme Q10, Calcium, Magnesium, Manganese, Selenium, Sodium, Zinc, and Glutathione.

6. Wellbutrin/Zyban depletes: Vitamin B6, Vitamin C, Vitamin D, Coenzyme Q 10, and Sodium.

7. Remeron depletes: Vitamin B6, Vitamin C, Vitamin D, Coenzyme Q10, Calcium, and Sodium.

8. Effexor depletes: Vitamin B1, Vitamin B2, Vitamin B3, Vitamin B6, Vitamin B12, Folic acid, Vitamin C, Vitamin D, Coenzyme Q10, Calcium, Magnesium, Manganese, Selenium, Sodium, Zinc and Glutathione.

9. Risperdal depletes: Vitamin A, Vitamin B1, Vitamin B12, Biotin, Folic acid, Carnitine, Inositol, Vitamin C, Vitamin D, Vitamin K, and Calcium.

10. Zyprexa depletes: Vitamin A, Vitamin B1, Vitamin B12, Biotin, Folic acid, Carnitine, Inositol, Vitamin C, Vitamin D, Vitamin K, and Calcium.

11. Seroquel depletes: Vitamin A, Vitamin B1, Vitamin B12, Biotin, Folic acid, Carnitine, Inositol, Vitamin C, Vitamin D, Vitamin K, and Calcium.

12. Depakote depletes: Vitamin A, Vitamin B1, Vitamin B2, Vitamin B12, Biotin, Folic acid, Carnitine, Inositol, Vitamin C, Vitamin D, Vitamin K, Calcium, Magnesium, and Essential fatty acids.

This information alone should give you a clear indication of why your health and mental state is declining through the use of western medicine and why it is so important to heal with nutrition, especially if one has been under the extremely toxic so called medication of allopathic medicine.

As it clearly states, it completely depletes these nutrients from the system, which means no matter how much of a healthy lifestyle one were to lead alongside the use of any of these medicines, they would eventually deplete your system of these nutrients making your need for these medications even greater. Rendering you dependent on these substances in order to function, all the meanwhile creating an even greater imbalance of nutrients in your system making you need higher dosages and eventually leaving your system malfunctioning and in some cases even with deadly outcomes.

I personally with my level of consciousness do not see how any of these medications can be used responsibly with any scientific or biological awareness whatsoever, as they will only work to decline a persons overall state of health and well being. I think it is reckless and unconscious behavior and as we see more people awaken to the truth of this world, we can only hope more people realize that healing is a very personal responsibility and we should not leave it in the hands of strangers, big companies with vast financial interests deep in the lobbies of our governments and infrastructure.

I have myself been on several of these myself and I can only testify to the declination of my health and well being mind, body and spirit as my illness progressed and their treatment increased and I eventually had such an intolerable existence I chose to suffer without medication for a short period of time rather than keep tormenting myself with what society has deemed medicine and healing, by taking my own healing into my own hands I healed on my own. What the medical community and even family and friends could only deem a miracle, or several miracles. But to the aware mind, it is no miracle, it is science, biology and alchemy and anyone can do it, if they so choose, but it means giving up everything you have given your consensus to, all your beliefs about healing and to gather your will, muster up your courage and start honing your intent and practice balance in all of these.

Will, Courage, Intent are three components to building a warrior spirit that also builds you as you build it, so the more you invest in these 3, the more these 3 invest in you.

There are days still where I have to fight to gather will to cross the threshold and exercise, push myself, but by building energy and getting out I gather more and more energy, knowing when to rest is key and knowing when to move your body, never go more than 2 days without exercise, then it easily drops back and motivation falters as a result of your setbacks.

I never thought I would run for miles in order to stay in shape or to take care of myself, I have almost always hated my body and I have almost always hated physical exercise as that was the dominion of the jocks that tormented me day in and day out for years through elementary and middle school.

Bullying is a killer for self love and healthy body image and as part of the healing of the masculine I have come to find a great many of us also suffer from an unhealthy body image due to Hollywood. We should by all means care for our vessels and make sure not to get diabetes and cancer, but to love our bodies as it is, as we work on improving it's overall state is fundamental to not falling in the pitfalls of self pity and start sabotaging our progress. So many times I have ended up a few pounds backwards just because I went into my self pity and ate my feelings for a couple of days processing some old traumas. But I came to find that the comfort eating didn't comfort, not like running did. Running comforts me and boosts me and makes me fitter, happier, healthier, more productive and less aggressive. It keeps me from experiencing the extreme outburst that I can get when I feel violated and under a lot of stress. Using adaptogenic herbs to boost my hormone levels has really helped me be able to deal with a lot more stress and when I could afford the herbal regime I need, I had no relapse symptoms in any of my imbalances. They were all healing from the use of the herbs and as soon as my ex and I broke up and I no longer could afford the expensive herbs, I started losing hair again and I had to go back on government aid in order to pay for my own healing so I can heal others.

Now, I can afford my nutritional regime 100% and finish my book without having to worry about money, my health and my social life. In the end I could hardly afford a night out a week with my friends to boost my mood and a depression kicked in as a result of my decline in health. I had to get back to health.

ENERGY WORK AND PRANA BREATHING

As I have mentioned earlier in my story, I was initiated by spirit in terms of certain abilities making themselves known to me during a very pivotal time in my life. I had long been told that I would become a healer by many psychics, shamans and healers in my time. Two of which later came to have been some of the most important teachers I have had in my life, one a shaman that worked as a teacher at the same school as my mom, who also mentored my mom and my sister in consciousness the time he was there, as shamans naturally take the role of guiding in whatever layer of society they find themselves in.

He saw my totem animal the sabre tooth tiger, which gave me lots of strength to tap into throughout my life and reminded me of the ancient being I knew myself to be, beyond this life and beyond time itself. He helped my sister through her psychic awakening as a teenager, with very powerful dreams and a lot of powerful healing happened for her, for me and for us together. My mom, my sister and I have always healed closely and in my shamanic awakening and with my suicide attempts my father also joined me in healing years of neglect and abuse both ways as I became more and more abusive in my addiction and I have for a decade now worked to understand how I have hurt my family and how to heal those wounds that caused them, the energies that birthed them, sustained them and created our family dysfunctions, most of all, our communication breakdowns, the triangulation from narcissistic templates, the twisted stories that makes one question their mental faculties and make these mental distortions that lead to mental imbalances.

The list of patterns, programs and templates that have been worked on within my family unit for the sake of this bloodline is not small. And it most likely will be the same for you reading this book, endless dysfunctional traits passed down for centuries down through the bloodline. Everything of which, starts in energy, as does everything in this universe and so it can be healed energetically as well, in the sheet bodies.

Which gets me to my other mentor who taught me a lot about

energy work.

The other mentor was an alcoholics anonymous counselor, healer and eventually friend which I came to learn a lot from and receive lots of important energy work from, which kept my heart open and helped me stay true to myself and my healing.

I wanted to get sober so bad, but I had such torment in me I wanted to escape from, it simply wasn't time yet, I had not learned the things I needed yet and had to walk alone through the darkness one more time, but with me now, I had my knowledge of healing that I had soaked up from this mentor, wonderful friend and amazing healer. A love for peace was found through the energy healing I received from Arvid and his genuine investment into my well being and sobriety made me believe in the hearts of men once again. I knew there were good people out there, I just happened to be in the wrong circles time and time again at the wrong place at the wrong time getting lesson upon lesson upon lesson. The energy work shifted that for me and things started gradually going better for me, but every time things got better, my self sabotage would kick in and I would end up back on the drugs again or back in trouble with other criminals, the law or my family, or all of the above all at once. It all just kept escalating until my whole life was such a mess there was no other choice left but to change, or die from the endless chains of bad choices and life threatening events I'd part take in on a daily basis as a drug fiend. It gets to a point where you know it's not going to last very long if you keep doing whatever it is that you are doing that is obviously not working out for you. You have come face to face with yourself and it all starts unraveling, you can no longer run, no longer hide and no amount of any drugs work like they used to any longer and no fantasy world or escapism sustainable whatsoever any longer.

You have reached the zero point, wherever you go from there will shape the rest of your life, so make wise choices, calculated moves, thread lightly and walk the path of heart, making heart based decisions for yourself and your life will produce heart based outcomes and what you formerly knew as karma will no longer exist and you now produce your reality from a conscious and expansive co-creator mindset. You have become an initiate and will continue to go through initiations in a never ending process of alchemy for as long as you live, this process never ends, it only goes in cycles as we evolve with the cosmic clockwork.

So we must come to know what the process is and how best to navigate the process as we progress and come to know ourselves more and more and understand what stages in the alchemy we find ourselves and how to make best use of the energy and the process we are in, in order to crystalize our consciousness and create gold out the lead, removing the false self construct, retrieving the true self behind the programming.

The true self as the holy grail of our quest in alchemy, to be restored to our blueprint as we were intended to experience life and contribute to the vast expansion of consciousness on a cosmic scale. We are so much bigger than we realize, we play such a major role in the lives we touch and the webs we weave as conscious dream weavers from a higher self perspective are extremely intricate and cannot be called anything less than divine design. To find our rightful place in this cosmos is sacred, to live out our blueprint as intended is a sacred act and to offer the ourselves, the world and the universe our unique talents, traits, gifts and consciousness, is nothing short of divine. It is our birth right to live out this way, to be who we were meant to be, to live out our highest versions of ourselves and be a beacon for others to join us in living out their highest versions of themselves as well.

This is what Meridian Energetics and the work I have been trained by higher self and the warrior spirit to do an do for you, restore you to your original blueprint and through the removal of ancestral energy, align you once more with your highest potential. This is my gift to the world in my highest version of myself and it has taken me years to hone and perfect this gift that once started out as a curse, a curse of taking on other people's energies, illness, pains and working hard trying to transmute it all only to end up sick myself. Had I not discovered the major importance of solitude and restoration of my own energy, I would have most likely not been here with the health I have today, that much is certain.

Everything is energy, everything starts out as energy and ends up as energy and energy always goes in and out of form, it never disappears, it never dies.
With this understanding of energy, we can heal anything, in energy, even before it becomes physical in its etheric state or after it has become a physical manifestation of the imbalanced energy. In my experience both as someone very ill as well as an experienced holistic healer, I find attacking any predicament from 3 angles is the only holistic approach that will lead to healing, first correct the thinking, or re-program yourself or your clients thinking about the illness, most people are stuck in a loop and their story and need help to break out of that loop of telling and reliving the story. Second is to attack the illness in the body, healing herbs and nutrient dense foods, detox and boosting immune system is your best approach towards healing the physical body. Third is to correct and balance the energy, the spirit of the illness, the imbalance, the consciousness, the energy in your sheet bodies.
When it comes to the energy that produces these expressions of illness, it is in fact what is hereditary and not in the DNA itself, nothing is truly hereditary in DNA, but in energy only, from generation to generation, passed down in the etheric body.
The DNA is immaculate, perfect, can be reprogrammed and restored by a conscious co-creator at will as well. Consciousness is all it takes, the awareness that we can speak to our cells, communicate with our organs, glands and have a conscious relationship with our physical vessel is beyond most people these days under the veil of their drug induced, desensitized unconscious existence. Our pains are simply our bodies trying to make us more aware of how we treat our bodies, to encourage higher awareness about how we operate and care for these vessels, these intricate biological machines we have been bestowed by creator to be able to co-create our dreams, or nightmares, all depending on the definitions and beliefs we have stolen from others.

Energy flows where attention goes, meaning anywhere you

place your attention for longer periods of time, will receive energy and healing. By you gifting yourself the attention your body so desperately needs, the body given the right conditions in order to heal, will always heal, that is its job. That is its purpose and its blueprint and by you removing toxins and eliminating obstructions for healing, you heal at an enormous rate. In my healing I went through two phases, one were I became an ugly caterpillar and every image of how I used to look would only haunt me and remind me of how I had lost my appearance and vitality and the second one, where I was healing a bit more and started using old photos of myself of how I wanted to look again to hold the vision of my healing.

I think both were important, especially the coming to terms with where I was and how far back it was going to be to heal all this and then equally creating my own healing through the use of the imaginative faculty and seeing myself in my own vision of the highest version of myself I wanted to be.

When the imaginative faculty, the heart center and the sexual centers are aligned we co-create our reality so much faster and so more aligned with who we truly are as a soul rather than who we think ourselves to be as human beings. The right people at the right time, the endless synchronicity, the constant winks from the universe that you are just where you are meant to be and big things are on its way, a five course meal on the menu and there is also going to be a heavenly dessert, vegan of course and life seem to only have plenty more of those in store for you.

It becomes clear to you, who you are, your purpose for being here and the role you are to play out in the expansion of consciousness as we experience it on planet earth at this time.

You have come home, home to your true self and the true self has no competition, it holds tremendous freedom to just be yourself, to just be you and not care what people think, not be dependent on validation, not crumble under criticism and to hostile haters, as there will always be both support and resistance to your work if you are doing altering work.

Nobody likes change, yet change is the only constant in this universe and that in itself can be both a healing thought and a scary thought, nothing you have now lasts forever and nothing you lose is truly lost forever, surrender to this thought, of change, it means things will not remain how they are for better or for worse and the universe has a way of changing things for the better, it is always the case in my case. Every loss seems carefully aligned with a greater gain in the end somehow.

It is evolution after all. Evolution always seeks to improve and as we find ourselves awakening, we find ourselves at the forefront of evolution, as consciousness itself evolves through us, first and foremost the pioneers and trailblazers of human consciousness, then the collective tends to catch up with us after some resistance. The trailblazers always enter the portals first and then the others catch up, it seems to have always been this way and we see the 100th monkey syndrome at work within the evolution of consciousness, monkey see, monkey do and so it is our responsibility to share our consciousness and ideas that set apart from the learned thinking of the societal constructs and conditionings. We are taught what to think and not how to think in classic education systems and if you want to retrieve something unique from the cosmic mind, you will have to learn to think for yourself, in your own lanes, channeling your own source intelligence and higher self through your human filters.

The more belief systems and filters we remove the more organic our experience.

TRANSPERSONAL ALCHEMY

Everything moves in cycles, with the clockwork of the cosmos , our solar system and as the living blueprint of alchemy, we enter different stages of evolution in our maturing process as human beings, on a mental, emotional and spiritual level.

We go through initiations in life and for each initiation passed, one level up in consciousness, awareness, presence, radiance, well-being and spiritual contentment and bliss. This is not to say we don't feel sadness anymore as illumined beings, yes we do, it however means that we transmute the sadness that comes up as alchemists and spiritually accountable beings.

But we have known such a deep hell and torment of mind, body and spirit in our initiations of alchemy in the dark night of the soul, visiting the hell within our own psyche and through transmutation eventually discovering our heaven on earth.

But first we have to go through hell, as the path to heaven leads through hell.

The Dark Night Of The Soul is in alchemy terms, the blackening, the stage known in the ancient arts of alchemy as nigredo. The initial stage of the process of alchemy. Many experience this at an astrological phenomenon called Saturn Return, which occurs every 7 years in your astrological chart. You may have noticed at the ages of 7, 14, 21, 27, 35, 42, 49, 56 and so on, major transformational events are more often than not happening in your life around that time. This is the cosmic finger print of Saturn. The father energy of our solar system.

We often get diseases, people die, we change jobs, divorce our partner or being part of a big accident and other very pivotal life changing events, like births, weddings, a life changing soul mate or moving into a new house, travelling the world and so on and so forth. The transformational events usually happen in the currents of Saturnalian Energy and leaves us forever transformed, more often than not, for the better, evolution always seeks to improve, so it is the cosmic clockwork of the solar system moves the alchemy forward, fulfilling our blueprints and living out our soul's purpose.

With the various initiations brought forth by codes or transmissions of energy or both, with plant medicines, psychedelics, entheogens, spells, rituals, but most of all by blueprint, as the living blueprint of alchemy is becoming templated in humanity on a collective scale with the upgrade from a seven chakra system to a twelve chakra system being set by the many so called volunteers as Dolores Cannon mentions in her work.

As the template is set the people being templated are experiencing initiations and activations from the 12 chakra upgrades, it is not for the faint of heart to go through these changes and upgrades but there are many now who have gone through these changes and if you need help with any such spiritual, physical, mental, emotional matters, or all of the above, please know you are safe and there are many of us out there now who can help and guide you back to health, balance and well being and it all starts in the gut.

Food is alchemy and as a species, we are by nature frugivore as Dr. Robert Morse says, I tend to agree with Dr. Morse, he is a sound, grounded, light hearted, truth-speaking medically trained holistic doctor, who guides people away from allopathic and traditional western medicine and the synthetic drugs they use to treat symptoms temporarily. He guides people towards the God's pharmacy module, but more importantly he is a great advocate for raw living, or fruitarian lifestyle, which I myself aspire to a lot, but cannot always afford. But I agree with Dr. Morse's philosophies of life, his approach to the natural science and biology, his use of herbs and fasting, his wisdom about the lymphatic system and endocrine system has only come to enrichen my life as it has countless others in the online health community and beyond.

I discovered Dr. Morse through my dear friend and inspirational health coach , herbalist , nutritional advisor, soul alchemist, author and life changing spirit catalyst Owen Fox. I found Owen in the afterglow of my dark night of the soul.

In 2011, living on an island in the south east of Norway at "Verden's ende" or in English "The Ends of The World" which lays in the Oslo-Fjord, right outside of Tønsberg, Norway's oldest city.

I had just broken up with my fiancé at the time after some very violent episodes involving pills, powders and alcohol.

I had decided to stop eating meat found Owen and later Dr. Morse, which have both helped me tremendously to heal myself of countless imbalances the past seven years since I discovered them. After I came off the medication from the doctors in 2011, I have not been to the doctor for anything other than blood tests and I had to have some stitches in my right foot last summer.

But I have become my own physician and doctor so to speak, Healing myself with food, exercise and lucid living, being accountable for what I put in my body, who I keep in my field, which affects our energy and template transferences and etheric debris of various kinds. People are scanned thoroughly before allowed to enter this space in any way, my energy is my greatest commodity and I use it not only to assist my clients all over the world, but I also use it for my own magick in life and in order to create good magick, we have to have good energy.

Feeling good and creating a harmonious space around you is pivotal during your time in the Nigredo, this is a time of coming to know all your shadows and learning to love them.

In this part of the process it is very normal to wish to cocoon and isolate one's self as we are overwhelmed by extra sensory perception, hallucinations, auditory, visual and physical, I often felt like I was sunburned, when there was no sun and I had not even been outside the door, I was undergoing some major physical and metaphysical transformations.

Everything starts in energy, so once the energy was activated within me, the process of alchemy is initiated within and without and I started seeing immediate changes happen within and without that was not of a positive nature, I was so afraid, I thought I was going to die and if I didn't die, somebody most likely was going to kill me. I was horrified and tormented by my kundalini awakening, which had given me kundalini syndrome, Or schizophrenic symptoms in medical terms.

I faced my own darkness and in guilt and shame I just wanted to die, the voices were telling me to kill the dog, kill my mom, burn the house down or someone else was going to, I chose to kill myself instead, for hours I fought the demons of my own creation in my mind, the fears I had accumulated, the visions of possible timelines and realities I had seen in my awakening,

Until I woke up that pivotal morning, on the couch at my mother's house, with her asking me, "So do you want to live, or do you want to die?", in which I replied, "I want to live".

It was as if my heart, my spirit all of a sudden found the strength to live through any hell I was provided with as I had now already seen a hell I wish upon no man, not even my worst enemies. The 3 days and nights that I fought my own fears, my own demons, the wheels of karma, staying in my heart energy I found a vortex which made feel safe, I had awoken as a conscious co-creator, seeing instant karma happen before my very eyes and being shown my previous karma cleared through the awakening of the heart. I accepted my personal hell, my nigredo became easier to live through in the acceptance of my very own personal hell. Months went by and little by little I got better and better as time progressed and I kept exercising and eating what I considered right at the time. But had I applied then what I know now, I could have shortened my healing time with five years. Clearing the lymphatic system and optimizing the endocrine system is simply so fundamentally life changing and will leave any person who tries it feeling a completely new human being. If the bodies sewage system and hormone factory is out clogged and out of balance, the body and the mind does not thrive very well and medication and further decay is usually the result as western medicine more often than not ends up pushing us pills, rather than advocating nutrition or a herbal solution which would be so much more healthy to the patient, but health is not what they are selling.

My alchemy kept happening as I went from agoraphobia, to exposure to my fears, step by step, breaking down my anxiety by exposing myself to anything that gave me weird syncs, anything that gave me fears, anything that would provide growth as I just wanted to get out of the mental hell and spiritual cage I had created for myself, co-created for me, so I would go in search of myself, in search of my healing, my light, my music, my poetry, my writing, my contemplation and analytical landscapes I so dearly love to wander and philosophize about anything above and below the firmament of human perception. It was during this "dark" time in my life, I found my warrior spirit, my light and my force and my will and intent, my intuitive and imaginative force and how I create with these and how to become a better equipped accountable co-creator. The initiations passed moving us to the next test and next challenge, always another level, always another place to arrive at in this process of alchemy, as it seem to never truly end, only like energy, go in and out of form.

Taking us from the one stage, over into the other,

In an endless oroborous, eating its own tail, we too also seem to transform, shed skin as we transmute the old and embody the new, the new you lies in the death of the old, every death onto yourself you experience rebirths, a new you, closer and closer to your true self with each death. To your essence, crystalized in being, in mind, body and spirit, through the alchemy processes that you undergo with the movement of the cosmos, the clockwork of the solar system. As new tides from various planets usher in different changes and different energies to assist us in orchestrating our lives and soul's purpose, we grow in different aspects of ourselves and experience transpersonal alchemy.

The lead of your mind, body and spirit, turned to gold, perfecting the mental, emotional, physical, spiritual self and retrieving the original blueprint of who you are, who you always were intended to be, but the ancestral family templates, patterns, programs and societal disruptions and entanglements kept you from embodying.

But with the alchemy burning away everything that is not you,

The true self emerges from the ashes of all the programming, patterns and dysfunctional traits we have taken on since birth.

Transpersonal alchemy not only heals the individual, but it seems to have an effect on the entire bloodline, the location where they live in a radius of miles, more or less all depending on the radiance of the individual in question.

It affects the people near-by by them being templated with the living blueprint of alchemy, the dormant meridians activated, the dormant twelve chakra system activated, in other words the template of sacred union and becoming cosmic humans.

This means you are not only transmuting in the local area you are living, but you are activating other people's process of alchemy, ushering in their initiations, activations and transformations. This in turn will eventually have the entire planet in a spiritual process of alchemy, so there will be a natural place and need for those who have undergone these processes personally and we might stand to see great chaos and confusion and a great many in need of spiritual assistance, spiritual healing and holistic approaches to mental health, physical health and spiritual well-being as more and more awaken to the reality of medication, the importance of nutrition and how all the chemicals, fragrances, aromas and synthetic materials in just about everything in our society is disrupting the endocrine system. If we are the living blueprint of alchemy, then what is our laboratory? You guessed it, our physical vessel, our meat-suit machine with its glands, organs, hormones and chemistry. Various foods have various frequency, trying mono-diets will make you better equipped at tapping into a specific fruit or vegetables frequency, once I had only eaten mostly loquats or oranges for 3-5 days I started noticing how these specific fruits were speaking to my cells, to my organs and the different energy I would get from eating watermelon mostly, oranges mostly or loquats mostly and so on...

I began feeling even more how food affected me and also how addicted I was to flavor, texture and certain compositions of foods based in my culture and upbringing, like bread, cheese, cucumber, mayonnaise and a little shrub of curly parsley, which is a very traditional sandwich in my family.

I was staying with Owen Fox and his girl at the time, Izumi and they were both deep into their raw lifestyle and a daily healing agenda for their lives which clearly was working for them both and through my stay there I became increasingly inspired to lead a healthier lifestyle by the minute.

We ate mostly fruit about 90% and 10% salads and miso soups with fermented foods incorporated into salads and soups and twice a week we would have a splurge and buy olives, maybe some goat cheese.

Occasionally I would sneak of for a day and have a steak or a pizza at a local restaurant with a glass of wine, as I was also celebrating this stage in my life, having gone from a dark night of the soul spanning a decade into mental illness and fighting for my physical health and agoraphobia afraid to leave the house, to traveling on my own in foreign countries meeting people who inspired me to change my life and to heal myself with herbs and nutrition as I had discovered partially myself,

But once I found just how much nutrition affects our mood, our longevity and wellness there simply was no going back.

It would be a severe case of cognitive dissonance to know the things I knew and not do anything about it. But with the level of food addiction I had a transition was also in order to not make me crave the bad foods I was used to, like chocolate, potato chips and other degenerative foods. Foods will either spark our cells and regenerate them like nutrient dense and rich foods or not and our cells are in constant decay suffering from the food-like products.

With Owen's inspiration and guidance I changed my lifestyle that spring and ate more fruit in a few weeks than I had been a whole year and it started showing on my skin, in my eyes and my hair and on the scale. When I came to the canary islands,

I weighed about 220 pounds from my more western lifestyle and I was very fatigued and exhausted from the process I was in as well as my body being very out of shape and beaten up from the drug abuse and suicide attempts. But I was determined to find a way to heal faster, especially to heal my erectile dysfunction, get the lymphatic system moving and to optimize the endocrine system. I knew if I could boost hormone levels and optimize the glands and organs my mental state, as well as my physical state would benefit highly. Boosting the adrenal after all those years of fight and flight mode in the criminal world, boosting the thyroid after all those years of drugs, the pancreas after all those years of sugars, the pineal and pituitary, boosting the kidneys and increasing filtration, boosting the liver. A year later I incorporated saunas, coffee enemas and parasite cures into my healing regime and experienced even deeper healing than I had before, emotionally as well as physically. I see it all as intrinsic and holistic, if I heal on spiritual level, the mind and body is affected, if I heal the mind, the body and spirit is affected and so on, so I have found my healing journey to work best for me covering my healing from a mental, emotional, physical, energetic, nutritional and spiritual approach covering all angles to be the best for me personally and it's a good advice to go at it from every angle in order to stop your imbalances in its progression.

Like I have mentioned before we are in fact at war for our consciousness, for our spirituality, for our life force, for our blueprint and purpose to come to fruition, for our health, our entire well-being and so the best strategy would be to increase our vitality, to boost our life force and live by blueprint,

It is the highest act of defiance in this unnatural world we inhabit. By living from our blueprint we actually hold the door for the natural world, the natural order of all things to sprout through the ground and blossom. By living from blueprint we stand in authenticity and in our authentic expression of self in our true self, we make it safe for others to be their true selves, it has a positive domino effect on other people and to be able to be ourselves fully, uninhibited and unafraid is needless to say,

Very healing to the mind, body and spirit.

With all the resistance to the natural expressions of who we are we create dissonance in our cells, we interrupt the natural harmony within our bodies, the frequency in our cells changing from the frequency of anxiety, from the frequency of fear, from the frequency of hate, constant anger and frustration, these frequencies are not good for our bodies and our cells over time.

They put us out of alignment with who we really are, what is meant for us may not find its way to us in our lives as we are so far away from who we intended for ourselves to be by design.

This is the reality for many people here on planet earth at this time and why so many are suffering, unhappy, unfulfilled, even and especially in the western world. They cannot find happiness as long as they don't know the true self, who they really are, their talents, gifts and reason for being here, it sets us free to simply be who we are, without restraints, without masks, simply be naturally, then everyone would find their rightful place, life by the natural order of the cosmos and fit in by not trying to fit in at all. Just one of the many paradoxical natures of this multiverse we find ourselves in.

My transpersonal alchemy includes so many things, but the most important factors for change has been diet and exercise, Herbs, nutrients and moving the lymphatic system have been the 3 most important components for my spiritual welfare and still to this day, they are part of my daily healing agenda.

However I would not have been so disciplined and able to parent myself as well, had it not been for the transformational work I did with Mel Brand healing my inner child, completing the merge of the masculine and feminine within and healing my emotional body and starting on healing the mental body with Meridian Energetics and meditation.
Healing the emotional body lead me to mature in ways I had found difficult until then due to triggers in the emotional body, wreaking havoc on my personal life, relationships and how I handled life. Living without constant triggers lead me to have more self-control and be better at distributing my energy, consciousness and time unlike anything I had experienced before and stealing my energy and triggering me into reaction mode nearly becoming impossible. I felt free and lighter than I ever had felt in my life, no longer would I be controlled by my reactions, or be such an easily triggered individual.
Able to conduct myself with more poise and presence in life and remain more in my peace, which over the years became my greatest commodity. Peace meant healing, peace meant restoration and rejuvenation. Peace meant bliss. It has become increasingly far in between the moments I am willing to give up my peace which has in turn made me more peaceful and my life more peaceful as a result.

Healing the mental body happens faster in peace, in silence, I often spend up to 5 hours in complete silence throughout my day, no music, no TV on, I find great peace in silent contemplation and nothing to distract me from what I am creating in this moment. Distractions from the true self are many and in our faces constantly in society from the moment we wake up to the moment we go to bed the matrix of our society is right there constantly grabbing at our attention, watering down our attention, our intentions, our intent and awareness, implanting thoughts and ideas about our inadequacy from our lack of looks, technological advancements, the latest car extravaganza or boat, coat, shoes, hairstyle, body shape, movie release, book release, music album release, concerts, festivals, TV shows, fashions, celebrities, the latest flavors, brands, from the ins and outs of popular culture to warfare and political drama, financial drama, rents, bills, schools, work, the worries are many and the solutions are few and often in pill form. Pills for every problem in life, mentally, emotionally, physically and even spiritually, there is a pill for every aspect of our lives in desperate need of healing.

Cultivating our own consciousness and reprogramming our mental body to think for us in constructive ways and not destructive ways as it has been by society, is of utmost importance if we are to co-create from our blueprint.

My dark night of the soul was extensive and the transformations in my transpersonal alchemy also extensive, Some would even say it is a miracle. And it is, it is a miracle that I am alive, it is a miracle that my mind still works to such an extent I can present these ideas and experiences to you all in such a fashion.

As the time spent in the underworld was so long for me, I had no choice but to surrender to the process and accept my own hell. A girl I was with a few years ago who said it quite well, In norse mythology we went to Hel in the underworld to get whole in mind, (Hel I Vettet – Norwegian). Odin hung himself upside down on the tree of life, Yggdrasil, with his mind in Hel, rooted himself in heaven, something which entirely fits the alchemical processes we see in the nigredo stage, the blackening. With Putrification we have everything putrid within us come to the surface to be released, in this stage I would often smell Sulphur even in the room and on my body, on my breath even. With a little bit of research there was clear to me an alchemical process was going on and the next step was to find ways to make the process more conscious and not be an unconscious spectator to my own spiritual process, but a conscious co-creator of my own spiritual process and facilitate a more conscious alchemy of mind, body and spirit.

I have since come to use the herbs, tinctures, minerals, vitamins and elements more consciously and produced results on a more conscious level. Knowing which herbs assist the various glands and organs and using nutrition and herbs consciously to assist the body in healing itself and creating healthy cell regeneration has been fundamental for my healing.

I strongly suggest you fall in love with learning about our plant kingdom and how to heal naturally alongside nature as it is the fastest way to heal I have found. The more natural I got the quicker I healed, it is not to deny. Nature heals everything.

Know thyself, is probably the most important alchemical phrase, as much as I AM is probably the most important magickal phrase, what we put after I AM shapes our reality after all, Abradacabra, I create what I speak.

But to create well, to truly know what to put after I AM,

We have to know ourselves. I AM sick, or, I AM healing,

Words are spells, that is why they call it spelling.

But I digress, the phrase Know Thyself, you have to know your self to love yourself and you have to love yourself in order to stop self sabotage and self destructive patterns in your ancestral bloodline. We carry so much that is not even ours to begin with, it is handed down energetically through our upbringing, through our conditioning and programming, through our ancestral patterns, through societal programming and templating. We have to know who we are, to know who we are not and vice versa, so we get lessons in what we are not to understand more of who we are. The more we experience things we do not want, the more we will realize we are not in alignment with who we truly are, our gifts, talents, traits, in fact our very blueprint remaining hidden due to our role in society, traumas and wounds, often from generation to generation,

Wounds handed down, relived, over and over throughout the family tree. The great work we do in the alchemy, ends this cycle of abuse, torment and disillusion and the "why me?"

victim mentality that often comes with generations of family members supposedly "born under an unlucky star", which of course is simply just another belief system, much like a curse will play itself out in a bloodline, due to belief, however so very very real to the family believing in curses.

Alchemy teaches us that the universe is mental,
In other words we create our experience of the universe from our mind, our definitions are human programs, our words are human programs and our labels, beliefs, religions, ideas and ideologies are all but human programs.
If we can change the way we define certain aspects and things in our lives, we can change the way we heal.
Change the way we manifest our illness or health,
lack or abundance, misfortune or fortune.
Our beliefs and definitions shape our reality,
Believing is seeing, not the other way around.
So you shape your reality from your belief system and experience your reality based on how you define and perceive your world. Once you break free of certain belief systems your entire world opens up, a new level of consciousness has been reached, yet your belief system has only been replaced by a new and upgraded belief system. We will always have belief systems as long as we operate within the third dimensional constructs of the human collective consciousness and its consensus reality,
Culture is the playground of human consciousness, where we get to lose ourselves and hopefully find ourselves, as we see more and more people are these days, losing themselves in a mindless job, finding themselves on a remote island, finding their way back to nature, to natural order, to natural living, natural healing and being naturally themselves, as they have started living from blueprint and have become the living blueprint of alchemy, in their true self, in their authentic soul expression. A spiritual beacon, through authentic embodiment inspiring others to embody more of themselves, to seek the self, to love the self and to live giving the gift of who we truly are.

You see, living from your blueprint, means leaving the mark on the world that you were intended to do before incarnation,

By design from your divine blueprint, this blueprint holds all the information of who you are as a soul, where you currently are at in your soul's evolution, all stored within the etheric body. Everything is energy, energy is information and frequency and everything has its frequency that it vibrates on. Everything vibrates, everything moves, nothing is truly solid.

You have non-physical bodies, called sheet bodies and in these sheet bodies are stored all the templates, patterns, programs and ancestral wounds, covering up the true self. Removal of these can be done by someone with the understanding of the sheet bodies and once these are removed, layer by layer etherically, the true self starts emerging and take shape.

A new process happens, which may take days, months or even a couple of years for the true self to really be strong. Still I find I have to stalk the ways in which I sabotage myself, my weaknesses as well as my strengths to not lose focus and let myself become my own worst enemy like so many times before. I have to be aware of who I am, to be who I am meant to be, I have to know myself. Knowing myself deeply, makes me able to know others more deeply and I can only be a good healer through healing myself. It all starts with self. Someone who is not aware of their own energies, will not be able to tune well into others energies and adjust them.

Energy work has become one of my greatest passions, to know I can assist someone in transmuting pain, hurt, suffering or just free someone from a stagnant personal evolution, assist them with health, diet, spirituality and make their world better, That is what I live for, why I came here. This is my blueprint. Transpersonal alchemy starts in becoming aware of our own shadow, or in layman terms "our own shit", but we don't stay there, we don't remain in the underworld of our psyche, through the progression of various stages of alchemy, we enter certain phases with glimpses of our true self, with deepening spiritual connection to nature, source, animals, people and the cosmos.

We come to find moments of clarity, stepping into lucidity, Living in a waking dream we come to recognize ourselves as dreamweavers. Conscious dreamweavers weave and manifest their reality with higher self, conscious dreamweavers are no longer participating in the nightmare known as culture in the same fashion as the people in slumber to the truth of everything. The truth is, none of this is real, it is all a dream and you are the dreamer, the dream being dreamt into being and in other words the director of your own movie, the writer, the lead actor, some of the cast, some of us even make the soundtracks to our own movies, which was always how I saw myself making music, adding music to my biography, my movie.

The hardest part for me to transmute has been the bullying and sexual abuse, the bullying festering in my psyche telling me I am not worthy of love, the sexual abuse festering in my psyche telling me I am not worthy of pleasure. Stifling my voice from singing out loud in the frequency of my true self, my soul song, how I harmonize with my cosmos unto myself and always did.

I stopped singing out of fear, I stopped dancing out of lack of joy, I stopped being me fully as all of me seemed too much for the world to handle and yes, while I was always intense and a lot, it was my talents, gifts and looks I experienced jealousy, envy and even hatred over. People hating you for simply being you, with decades of that kind of energy directed at you, you will eventually either become a warrior or a victim.

Many children and teenagers commit suicide for even half of what I went through in my childhood and early teen years.

The saddest part is they learn it through their parents and media, media constantly bullies, slanders and runs celebrities down to the ground, the collective unconscious loves to pick people apart and we are programmed to measure ourselves and others to ridiculous standards that not anyone can meet, so we all walk around feeling inadequate and misplaced, not knowing we are perfect just as we are and beauty is in the eyes of the beholder and not set by popular culture which is often digitalized, edited, drugged down versions of reality with the intent of making artificial beauty the standard so we all feel like we are not enough. I am currently working on my first music album release and the voices in the back of my mind from the bullying are still there, but I choose not to listen, I love myself too much to allow anyone to hold me down, hold me back or keep me from my victories that I have fought so hard for spanning decades now. I crave my blueprint, yet at the same time, the true self is large, larger than life and to embody the true self, we ourselves become truly larger than life as well, as we transcend life in our defiance of death, decay, delusion and disillusionment, we hold something bigger than even life itself. We hold source code blueprint, source creative energy authentically expressed working as a transmutation activator and transfiguration coordinator simply through the embodiment of the true self, as the living blueprint of alchemy.

Source creative energy is sexual energy, it is your life force, your chi, your vitality, the amount of source creative energy you are able to conduit and channel is in direct relation to the health of your endocrine system, or in other words your chakras.

The healthier your organs and glands the stronger your chakras and vice versa, the chakras are the energy centers for the organs and glands and the meridians flowing through your limbs and the etheric body works as tubes for the energy coming in and out of the etheric body and your physical body. We can remove something physical energetically and we can remove something energetic physically, in my healing work I have found it detrimental to go at the illness from all angles, mind body and spirit. So how I think about the illness, my mental experience of the illness, then my body, what my body needs facilitated to rejuvenate, regenerate and restore itself, then I look at the energy behind the illness, where it is stored and remove the illness, layer by layer in the sheet bodies.

Health has to be found in the holy trinity to be holistic and lasting, there has to be a seed planted in the mind to change the thinking that created the dis-ease in the first place, then the actions that lead to our dis-ease, what we put in our bodies, how we maintain our vessels and to finally become sovereign beings, knowing ourselves, knowing nature, nutrition and how to facilitate healing well enough ourselves to become our own doctors. Our way of living has become a healing experience all of itself and not by coincidence, but by design, by blueprint.

The living blueprint of alchemy affects everything it comes into contact with, activating and templating others to start their process in retrieving their very own blueprint. This is our work. Paracelsus is an alchemist that has fundamentally changed my life for the better and made me able to see my own process of alchemy and purification in a very concise and simple to understand and presented in a holistic light. So in this chapter we will look at the seven rules of Paracelsus and how you can use them to heal your own life and facilitate simple, yet profound alchemy in your own mind, body and spirit.

THE SEVEN RULES OF PARACELSUS

(For a successful alchemical process)

Paracelsus (/ˌpærəˈsɛlsəs/; late 1493 – September 24, 1541), born **Philippus Aureolus Theophrastus Bombastus von Hohenheim**, was a Swiss German philosopher, physician, botanist, astrologer, and general occultist. He is credited as the founder of toxicology. He is also a famous revolutionary for utilizing observations of nature, rather than referring to ancient texts, something of radical defiance during his time.

He is credited for giving zinc its name, calling it zincum.

Modern psychology often also credits him for being the first to note that some diseases are rooted in psychological conditions.

Paracelsus' most important legacy is likely his critique of the scholastic methods in medicine, science and theology. Much of his theoretical work does not withstand modern scientific thought, but his insights laid the foundation for a more dynamic approach in the medical sciences.

Paracelsus hermetical views were that sickness and health in the body relied on the harmony of Man (microcosm) and Nature (macrocosm). He took a different approach from those before him, using this analogy not in the manner of soul-purification but in the manner that humans must have certain balances of minerals in their bodies, and that certain illnesses of the body had chemical remedies that could cure them. As a result of this hermetical idea of harmony, the universe's macrocosm was represented in every person as a microcosm.

An example of this correspondence is the doctrine of signatures used to identify curative powers of plants. If a plant looked like a part of the body, then this signified its ability to cure this given anatomy. Therefore, the root of the orchid looks like a testicle and can therefore heal any testicle associated illness. Paracelsus mobilized the microcosm-macrocosm theory to demonstrate the analogy between the aspirations to salvation and health. As humans must ward off the influence of evil spirits with morality, they also must ward off diseases with good health.

Paracelsus believed that true anatomy could only be understood once the nourishment for each part of the body was discovered. He believed that therefore, one must know the influence of the stars on these particular body parts. Diseases were caused by poisons brought from the stars. However, 'poisons' were not necessarily something negative, in part because related substances interacted, but also because only the dose determined if a substance was poisonous or not. Paracelsus claimed the complete opposite of Galen, in that like cures like. If a star or poison caused a disease, then it must be countered by another star or poison. Because everything in the universe was interrelated, beneficial medical substances could be found in herbs, minerals and various chemical combinations thereof. Paracelsus viewed the universe as one coherent organism pervaded by a uniting lifegiving spirit, and this in its entirety, Man included, was 'God'. His views put him at odds with the Church, for which there necessarily had to be a difference between the Creator and the created.

Realizing I had used much of Paracelsus formula from intuition and guidance from the higher self, I started using his formula more consciously and I quickly began to experience fundamental changes in my psyche, in my physique and my energy, many of my clients reporting back even stronger reactions to my energy work and noticeable changes within my work, writings, my appearance and as I started excavating the true self from the rubble of cultural conditioning and ancestral programming I realized I was now ready and able to assist others in a much more profound manner and as I am in this writing moment breeching a writer's block to finish my book, I come to find myself in yet another place of being able to gift others the gifts that I give myself through arduous and exhausting, but oh so rewarding soul work. Through my alchemy studies I also came across two amazing alchemists, Dennis William Hauck and his great work and Avery Hopkins and his great work. Both laboratory alchemists as well as spiritual alchemists, I added their great work to my process and through using other great alchemists who came before me I made my own process of alchemy easier.

As I now look outside the firmament with true cosmic consciousness, I find everything under the stratosphere to be of human construct and belief systems, even sciences like alchemy and astrology to even be belief system tools that I can play with in my human experience. An experience is never free from the belief systems the experiencer holds, in other words we shape our reality from our beliefs. This holds us in incredible accountability as it makes us the co-creators of our reality, of our experience of life. We can no longer blame anyone else for how we fail in life, where we are at, where we are going, is entirely up to us and so we start making the changes necessary to heal our lives and we mature mentally, emotionally and spiritually. If you were truly of cosmic consciousness you would not give your power away to ascended masters, archangels and angels, ancient avatars, deities of any kind or a messiah. You would know these as archetypal energy that we have created as a collective consciousness under the dome or the firmament. Something that I came to understand through experience as well as the great work of Carl Gustav Jung and his extensive work on transpersonal alchemy.

How can I say such a thing? Well, most of what we experience here on earth is not defined and experienced in the same way on other planets, systems throughout the multiverse as they have their ways of defining reality, their definitions, labels and understanding from their individual and collective consensus and perception of reality.

When you truly come to understand this, you are free, there is no longer anything to defend, anything to fight over, there is no enemy and only victims of unconsciousness, or warriors in the game. We cannot be both, one will eventually destroy the other and we either come out defeated or as victors of our own transformation as a result of a strong warrior spirit.

The warrior spirit came to life in full force within me during my kundalini awakening and it has both challenged me, changed me, healed me as well as put me in danger of death.

The higher self, or the warrior spirit, will go to any great lengths in order to get you to where you need to be, spiritually.

It will even put you in a car accident, remove people from your life, remove your job, your home, give you a lethal illness or other challenges for you to step out of who you were and who you were becoming, to get you to become who you were always meant to be. You may be reading this book right now feeling in deep resonance with these words and it is no accident this book found its way to your hands and sharing my experience with you here in book format, is part of my deprogramming of your mind, my contribution to your freedom, free of the matrix constructs, free of disillusionment from the health industry and free of the confusion of dis-ease. I wish for you to find your health, I wish for you to be free of so called medication from the doctor, I wish for you to thrive, to embody your true self and feel at home in creation, to claim your rightful place in creation as all that is would not be all that is without the puzzle piece that is you. So don't cut yourself short, don't water yourself down and most of all, love yourself enough to allow yourself to live the life you always wanted. Invest in who it is you wish to become daily. As a line of direction, I use Paracelsus model to keep my daily healing agenda at a simple, yet profound track to optimal health and spiritual well being.

If you would like to dive deeper into understanding the stages of transpersonal alchemy, I highly suggest you read Dennis William Haucks book "The Emerald Tablet".

But even implementing Paracelsus 7 rules, I had enough of a transformation that I realized I was on the road to success.

And two years later, I am still a work in progress to perfect it, but as my mentor and friend Mel Brand says, perfectly close will do. Sticking to it daily 90% of the time and 10% of indulgence has lead me to experience profound alchemy in my own life. I am in better shape now than I was when I was in my early twenties as I was never very into running and exercise, something that has changed with my process of alchemy and my wish for optimal performance of mind, body and spirit.

~ THE SEVEN RULES OF PARACELSUS ~

1 • The first is to improve health. This is to breathe as often as possible, deep and rhythmic, with well-filled lungs, be outside or looking out a window. Drink in small sips every day, two liters of water, eat lots of fruits, chewing food as perfect as possible, avoid alcohol, snuff and medicine, unless for some reason you were subjected to severe treatment. Bathe daily is a habit that you owe to your own dignity.

2 • Absolutely banish from your spirit, for many reasons that may exist, any idea of pessimism, resentment, hatred, boredom, sadness, revenge and poverty.
Run away like the plague of every opportunity to treat people cursing, vicious, vile, murmuring, lazy, gossipy, vain or vulgar and inferior natural baseness of understanding or sensualist topics that form the basis of their speeches or occupations. The observance of this rule is of decisive importance: it's about changing the spiritual texture of your soul. Is the only way to change your fate, because this depends on our actions and thoughts. The chance does not exist.

3 • Do all the good possible. Help all unhappy people whenever you can, but never have any weaknesses for any person. You

take care of your own energies and flee from all sentimentality.

4 • Forget all offense, more over: strive to think well of your greatest enemy. Your soul is a temple that should never be desecrated by hate. All the great beings have been guided by this gentle inner voice, but it won't speak to you like that all of a sudden, you have to prepare for some time, destroying the overlapping layers of old habits, thoughts and mistakes that weigh on your spirit, which is divine and perfect in itself, but impotent so imperfect vehicle that you offer today to demonstrate , lean meat.

5 • You have to retire each day where no one can bother you, at least for half an hour, sit as comfortably as possible with your eyes half closed and think of nothing. This strengthens strongly the brain and the Spirit and puts you in contact with good influences . In this state of meditation and silence, bright ideas tend to occur , capable of changing an entire existence. Eventually all the problems that arise will be resolved victoriously by an inner voice guiding you in these moments of silence, alone with your conscience. That is the daimon of Socrates speaking.

6 • You maintain absolute silence of all your personal affairs. Abstain, as if you've made a solemn oath, to relate to others, even your most intimate, whatever you think, hear, know, learn, suspect or discover. for a long time at least you should be as a walled house or a sealed garden. It is a rule of utmost importance.

7 • Never fear men or inspire you fright the DAY of tomorrow. Keep your mind sharp and clean and you will do well. You never feel alone or weak, because there are powerful armies behind you, which you cannot conceive even in dreams. If you raise your spirit there is no evil that can touch you. The only enemy you should fear is yourself. The fear and distrust in the future are dire mothers of all failures, they attract bad influences and with it disaster. If you study carefully people of good luck, you'll see that intuitively they follow a great part of

the rules above. Many of those who achieve richness, it is very true that they are not quite good people, in the strict sense, but have many virtues mentioned above. Moreover, wealth is not synonymous of happiness, it may be one factor that leads to it becuse of the power that gives to exercise great and noble work, but more lasting happiness can only be achieved in other ways; There where the old Satan of the legend never reigns , whose real name is selfishness. Never complain about anything, dominate your senses, flee both humility and vanity. The humility takes strength from you and vanity is so harmful that it is like saying: a mortal sin against the Holy Spirit.

~ PARACELSUS

Much of the importance of Hermeticism arises from its connection with the development of science during the time from 1300 to 1600 AD. The prominence that it gave to the idea of influencing or controlling nature led many scientists to look to magic and its allied arts (e.g., alchemy, astrology) which, it was thought, could put Nature to the test by means of experiments. Consequently, it was the practical aspects of Hermetic writings that attracted the attention of scientists.

Taken from Wikipedia

Implement these practices of Paracelsus into your life and watch your life transform, it is that simple, yet it is hard for many, due to programming and addictions, but if I can do it, anyone can. I am in this writing moment finally entering my coagulation in the process of alchemy.
I am at a place in my journey that seems rather raw, fresh and treading new ground, breaking personal barriers and personal bests in my private life, my book is almost done, my soul work almost ready to be released to the world and I feel confident in who I am, what I am delivering and the 10 years it took me to get to where I am today. 10 years after the spiritual awakening

that scared me straight and put me on the straight and narrow path, doing Karma yoga to make up for the hardship I had imposed on others through my drug addiction.

I am no longer an addict, I no longer smoke 10 cigarettes a day or pop pills and all kinds of drug cocktails to sustain my need for connection.

That is all addiction really is, need for connection.

I can enjoy just about anything now without letting it consume me entirely, as I am aligned and connected. I now navigate life easier and I can live my life in a balanced way, thanks to the healing work I have done and the many, many mentors that have helped me on the way here.

I didn't get here alone. I made alliances.

I got here thanks to blood, sweat and tears,

deep bonds and love from my family and friends along the way and then there were teachers that showed up at just the right time, to help me elevate,

I could have scoffed them off with my ego, but I reveled in their teachings in the depths of my being and my heart connected deeply with them all and a part of them all lives on inside of me.

Their words and presence.

To have been blessed with such huge teachers as I have been is not many bestowed and I am well aware of the force of those who came before me,

which also lives within me, we attract what we are,

to help us become what we are meant to become.

Where you are right now, is exactly where you need to be.

Whether it is lessons or blessings or a mix of both,

You are in this very moment as part of who you are becoming.

If you don't like who are becoming, change the script, change location, cast, whatever you need. You are the director of your life, you are the one navigating the challenges and the opportunities that arises,

Nobody else.

Life happens to us and through us, sometimes we can't help but go through some traumatic experiences,

But we can choose to let them make us kinder, softer and yet tougher at the same time as we learn to deal better with our own and others shit.

Not everything makes sense as it transpires, but once it all settles and the dust clears we find treasures within the most hurtful events.

Don't let life make you bitter, Become better.

That is what the world needs more of, kind, loving people.

And the alchemy of life, has a tendency to make us softer, eventually, we all face ourselves.

And in an instant, we are forever changed.

Alchemy, this process many of us find ourselves in consciously or unconsciously, is meant to polish us into better beings.

It is meant to create gold from the lead of our being.

The alchemists most profound tool in creating himself as a God/Co-Creator, is his or her imaginative faculty.

That partnered with a fully operational heart center that has been activated over and over through various stages of soul alchemy, creates what the alchemist needs to finish his great work and bring it back into the world.

This is the final stage of his alchemy.

His Coagulation.

The circle is complete.

Solve Et Coagula.

As the amazing alchemist and author, Dennis William Hauck mentions in his book, The Emerald Tablet, "The tarot cards symbolizing Coagulation are paradoxical, the devil and the magician/hierophant, who is making his second appearance as Hermes Trismestigus in the process, earlier appeared during Fermentation and now in Coagulation. Together the Hierophant and the Devil stand for the opposing forces of light and darkness that come together in the higher marriage, the marriage of heaven and hell, which produces the divine androgyne, or the stone. The Androgyne often showing as a boy, mercury, Symbolizes the joining of the opposites on all levels necessary at this stage."

"In this state of clarity, the alchemist knows exactly who he is, what he believes,
and what is going on within him at any given moment. The newly discovered presence from his coagulated being becomes a permanent stone, which he can rely on and touch any time he pleases."

He goes on to explain further in his book,
"Before the Coagulation occurs in a person, he or she can appear to be arrogant or self-involved because of their preoccupation with finding perfection and divinity within themselves. Afterwards, the exude a unique presence, a steady confidence in their daily activities, and others begin to see them as authentic and whole persons whom they want to emulate. People sense this higher presence and want to worship it, he says, which sometimes results in the quasi religious following of Balinas and Alexander the great. Modern examples are Ramana Maharishi and Parmahansa Yogananda, and mystics like George Gurdijeff, who have huge followings worldwide."

I am also experiencing all of this alchemy in alignment with the planets, my Jupiter return is coming up and lots of Leo and sun energy directing me to take my place in the sun, to claim what is mine from the work I have done. But how the planets affect my alchemy is something I am sure we will get back to in another book, or in my future work as it is highly fascinating to see the patterns in life unfolding in alignment with the planetary cycles.

This stage of the alchemy is rightfully earned and I am now a self-made man, a story of victory, over my own demons,
over many addictions, over illness and mental illness.
Years of suffering, hard work and studying mysticism and alchemy, astrology, psychology, herbs, energy healing modalities and human anatomy.
In order to claim my own health and happiness and offering others a chance to find theirs, through what is my great work,

Holistic mental health.
I tend to go off radar for a while as I love to go inwards during these shifts,
but I will be available for sessions and writing articles in the time to come, but if you want to read more of my free work and articles, you will have to come to my website,
So stay tuned, for the fruits of my coagulation.

Dear Soul Family, Clients, Family and Friends,
thank you for all the love and support over the years,
and to YOU reading this very book right now,
thank you for having the courage to finish this ride with me,
you all mean the world to me.

Much love,

Ulf Haukenes

ABOUT THE AUTHOR

Ulf Haukenes is an etheric surgeon, holistic healer, nutritionalist, poet, musician, writer of metaphysical content for many years. He has published many articles for the twin flame community on metaphysical concepts from his shamanic awakenings and continue to do so to this day. He has successfully assisted and guided many through their spiritual awakenings and healing crisis and healed himself from countless diagnosis given to him by western medicine, including severe diagnosis such as bipolar disorder, borderline personality disorder, schizoid personality disorder as well as depression, anxiety, panic attacks related to C-PTSD, malnutrition, auto immune disorders such as alopecia universalis and less severe ones such as obesity, lethargy and more. Apart from his ongoing spiritual awakening he is a herbalist, botanist and alchemist and you can find his writings and videos all over the online spiritual community.

His vision is to assist as many as possible to thrive in mind, body and spirit.

Made in the USA
Middletown, DE
21 August 2021

46609355R00066